LIVING PAIN FREE

The Alleviate Way

DR. SWAGATESH BASTIA

STARDOM BOOKS

www.StardomBooks.com

STARDOM BOOKS
A Division of Stardom Publishing
and infoYOGIS Technologies.
105-501 Silverside Road
Wilmington, DE 19809

FIRST EDITION JULY 2022

STARDOM BOOKS

A Division of Stardom Alliance
105-501 Silverside Road Wilmington, DE 19809,
USA

www.stardombooks.com

Stardom Books, United States
Stardom Books, India

LIVING PAIN FREE
The Alleviate Way

Dr. Swagatesh Bastia

p. 237
cm. 13.5 X 21.5

Category:

MED093000 - Medical : Pain Medicine
HEA036000 - Health & Fitness : Pain Management

ISBN: 978-1-957456-09-6

DEDICATION

To anyone who is suffering from chronic pain or watching their
loved ones facing the challenges of chronic pain.

To those who have tried various sporadic treatments to no effect
and those who have accepted chronic pain as a peril of aging.

This book would have served its purpose if it helps the readers take
even one positive step in the direction of getting better

PREFACE

Having spent almost a decade in the practice of Orthopedic Surgery, there are some questions that keep troubling me often. The most pertinent of these are concerning the patients coming to the orthopedic OPD for a consultation. On average, only 2 to 3 people out of 20 seen in the ortho clinic are patients with proper indications to undergo orthopedic surgery. When orthopedic surgeons identify and diagnose an operable case, this becomes the center of their attention as they are keen to bring about a positive impact on the concerned patient's quality of life with their surgical skills. And they know they can do it.

My problem was this: Patients suffering from chronic pain for years due to non-operable causes, such as early arthritis, tendonitis, partial ligament injuries, and sacroiliac joint dysfunction, would pass under the radar as innocuous. Looking for relief from chronic pain, they would consult numerous doctors and medical practitioners, who would prescribe myriad medications and kinds of physical therapy. Despite reassurances from the doctors, they often do not obtain relief from their pain, and slowly but surely, the patient starts turning captive to the vicious circle of chronic pain.

After spending a couple of years traveling around America and Europe, spending time in Pain and Regenerative Clinics, I came to the conclusion that an 'INTEGRATED PATIENT-CENTRIC MULTIDISCIPLINARY APPROACH' was the answer to the management of chronic pain.

At Alleviate, we are trying to do exactly the same on the Indian subcontinent in order to improve the quality-of-life index of as many people as possible. Through this book, I want to spread awareness about chronic pain and spark the desire to get better in those suffering from chronic pain.

CONTENTS

ACKNOWLEDGMENTS

My sincere acknowledgments go out to my family for their
continued support and encouragement to go through my first
writing expedition.
I thank our Nutritionist, Ms. Pooja Shankar, and our Clinical
Psychologist, Ms. Sonam Manoj, for their valuable contributions to
the chapters on 'The Role of Nutrition' and 'Clinical Psychology,'
respectively.

1

VICIOUS CIRCLE OF CHRONIC PAIN

"Numbing the pain for a while will make it worse when you finally feel it."
– JK Rowling in Harry Potter and The Goblet of Fire

Pain is something we all universally try to avoid. Pain is associated with negativity and stress. It is generally considered undesirable. We think, there could possibly be no benefits from pain. But is this true? JK Rowling's statement is quite the fact when we talk about the pain experienced in our bodies—physical pain. Pain in any part of our body tends to serve as an indicator that something is wrong and needs to be checked out immediately. Ignoring pain when it first occurs can lead to severe consequences as we will see through the chapters of this book.

So, we can all agree that acute pain serves a good purpose. Sometimes, owing to negligence or other causes, people suffer from chronic pain. Chronic pain is defined as pain that persists in a tissue or organ of the body past the normal healing time.

Pain

More changes in
the nervous system

Anxiety that pain
is signalling tissue
damage and harm

**Chronic
Pain Cycle**

More anxiety and
less movement

Brain becomes
more focussed
on the problem

More Pain

Changes
take place in
the nervous
system

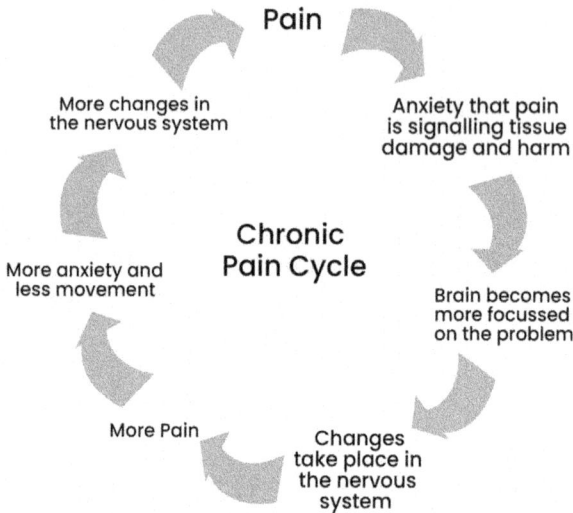

Chronic ailments like hypertension, diabetes, and thyroid disorders have been accepted by society as agents with substantial potential for threat to good health. They have been studied and researched for many decades, and today we are blessed to have excellent treatment protocols for each of these. On the other hand, chronic pain is perceived by many as something innocuous, a peril of aging, or even as an inevitable companion for the rest of their lives. People do not realize that chronic pain soon makes itself comfortable and starts its vicious circle of harm, and in no time, it is defeating the host in the everyday battle of life!

As you can see from the list of pains and conditions discussed later in the book, chronic pain literally resides in every household. Studies have shown that approximately 30 percent of people across populations are suffering from chronic pain at any given point in time.

Though it has a preponderance for old age, the heightened daily stress levels in today's multifaceted lives have enabled chronic pain to make its presence felt in the lives of young adults as well.

Chronic pain ushers a wave of negative emotions like anxiety, fear, and an overbearing omnipresent feeling of being unwell. The growing anxiety is fueled by increasing pain, which in turn keeps alerting the brain to the ongoing tissue damage and harm. This makes the brain increasingly sensitive and focused on the pathology that induces changes in the nervous system leading to more pain and anxiety. As a result, the affected individual becomes less mobile and is caught deeper in the web of pain and anxiety!!

A person battling the vicious cycle of chronic pain uninterrupted over a period soon begins to lose motivation and underperform professionally, straining relationships and experiencing a gradual but imminent decline in happiness and quality-of-life index!

Usually, any pain lasting over three months is referred to as chronic pain. Chronic pain may be present continuously in certain conditions or it may be brought on by certain activities or actions, such as pain associated with arthritis. Some people are more sensitive to pain following certain illnesses or disease conditions, which caused some changes in the body. For example, patients who underwent radiation therapy to the chest wall can suffer from chronic pain in the ribs.

Sometimes chronic pain may not have an associated physical cause like an injury or illness. This kind of pain may be brought on by stressful conditions or anxiety. This is termed psychogenic or psychosomatic pain. Whatever the cause of chronic pain, it can lead to a lot of other distressing symptoms in the sufferer. Chronic pain leads to anxiety, depression, sleep disturbances, mood swings, etc. It can seriously affect the quality of life of the patients.

Therefore, it is important to identify the source of pain and treat it appropriately. There are various tests and investigations that can help in diagnosing chronic pain. Imaging modalities play an important role in the diagnosis of bone or joint-related pain. Depending on the diagnosis, doctors prescribe therapy to combat chronic pain. Apart from the use of medications, it has been proved that various lifestyle changes can effectively combat or decrease chronic pain.

People have benefitted from regular low-intensity exercise routines and meditation. Doctors have also recommended that getting adequate sleep can help in reducing chronic pain. Nutritionists recommend the inclusion of anti-inflammatory foods in the diet to help combat chronic pain. So, as you can see, there are various modalities of treatment to help a patient with chronic pain. But the will to get better must come from the patient. Having an attitude of fatality toward chronic pain prevents the patient from getting better.

Let us see what needs to be done from the patient's side in dealing with chronic pain.

First Step: A Will to Get Better

> *"To live without Hope is to Cease to live."*
> – Fyodor Dostoevsky.

In my practice, I have seen many patients who prefer not to undergo surgical therapy for chronic pain. I understand their point of view, and I would even commend it. The surgical option should be taken only when specifically indicated.

However, many patients with chronic pain choose not to consult a specialist at any point. And even when they do go for a consultation, they do not believe they can get better. I see this very often in our clinic. Patients accept pain as inevitable and they do not have any WILL to GET BETTER. They lack the will to undergo treatment, practice rehabilitation measures, or follow nutritional guidance. This is very important. The patient must be willing to break away from the shackles of old behavior. He/she must be willing to work with their healthcare provider toward healing and recovery. Lack of motivation over the years has rendered many a patient a reservoir of chronic pain. This is effectively due to years of tissue damage, poor dietary habits, faulty lifestyle choices, and neglect. Now what they look for is a QUICK FIX, an EASY FIX, and a PAINLESS FIX for their pain.

It is indeed true that there are treatments and medications that can help relieve chronic pain substantially and enable you to get on to the battlefield, but to achieve marked and lasting improvement in pain, you need to have the will to change your habits and better your lifestyle, not just for a day or two but forever.

Dear reader, if you are a person suffering from chronic pain and have been contemplating doing something about it for a long time, I would encourage you to cast the rope of WILL POWER into the well of denial, self-pity, and resentment that you have dug for yourself and climb out to avail the various treatment options that are available.

Second Step: Be Well-Informed

Once you have mustered the courage to deal with your chronic pain, the next important point to note is AWARENESS. You must become aware of your condition. You must learn all about your disease and the various treatment options that are available. This is one of the striking differences that I noticed when I practiced in England. There, the patients were more knowledgeable and informed about their pain and the management options than patients in India are. I believe that a good level of understanding of the condition causing you grief can go a long way in guiding you on the appropriate treatment path.

In my practice, I have come across patients with chronic pain who have been suffering for decades. They would have visited numerous doctors and tried numerous treatments such as medicines, massages, and oils for local application. But in all these years they would not have been given a DIAGNOSIS of their condition! Can you believe it?

In the present times, people undertake exhaustive background checks before purchasing an apartment or spend hours researching before deciding on which telephone model to buy. And when it comes to buying a car, I am truly amazed at the intricate details that people go into before making their ultimate choice!

It is not my intention to criticize those who make their choices with utmost care. Do not mistake me. But this is highly frustrating from a medical practitioner's point of view. How can you go on for years visiting doctors and specialists without asking for your diagnosis?

This is what I want to impress upon you, dear readers. This is my message, loud and clear—You have to ask for a diagnosis when you visit a medical practitioner or a specialist. Do whatever it takes; undergo the necessary tests and investigations. But ensure that you know what is ailing you.

Once you know your diagnosis, spend some time understanding your condition, read up about the relevant signs and symptoms, look up the various treatment options, and if there are friends or relatives who have had a similar experience, talk to them as well. Keep yourself well-informed. Find out who are the specialists who are experts in treating your condition.

Third Step: Seek Good Counsel

Identifying a doctor or specialist who is an expert in managing your condition can go a long way in your treatment. This will put you in a much better place and also allow you to make informed decisions about your treatment options and the course of management. The importance of having good counsel cannot be stressed enough. Getting reliable and good medical advice is essential for your recovery. The medical field is advancing rapidly and healthcare professionals need to keep pace with the developments. Your doctor must be someone who is up to date with the developments in his/her specialty.

We see so many patients in our clinic who have been misled by poor counsel. They have undergone unnecessary suffering and worsening of their condition over many years. Patients with conditions like fibromyalgia (Chapter 3) frantically search for anything that can give them a pain-free life. But the crucial aspect of diagnosis is missed and therefore they are denied appropriate therapy. They would have had numerous consultations with specialists through numerous referrals, only to be told that the pain is all in their heads. A diagnosis could have been arrived at if only the medical practitioner had taken the time to listen patiently to the patient and, more importantly, is aware of the condition of fibromyalgia.

This is immortalized in the words of Robertson-Davies, the Canadian author: *"The eye sees what the mind is prepared to comprehend."* Your doctor can diagnose a condition only when he knows about it and recognizes the signs and symptoms. That is why it is important to get wise and correct counsel for chronic pain! So, what is the solution? You have to find a specialist who is skilled in making the correct diagnosis.

You have to find a specialist who has a good track record in treating the condition. A good doctor will patiently listen to your story, discuss your condition at length with you, and explain in detail the various treatment modalities that are available. Let me tell you about one of our patients, Raman, who visited our clinic with chronic pain.

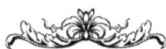

CASE STUDY 1

Raman was a 35-year-old software engineer who came to our clinic with chronic pain in his right ankle. He had been suffering from ankle pain for over a decade now. The pain had first come on following an ankle injury during a college football match.

At that time, he had been diagnosed to have had a sprain and advised to follow all the usual treatments for a sprain: pain medications, cold compress, the elevation of the foot, elastocrepe bandaging, etc. The acute pain subsided in a week or so, but over the years, Raman started having pain in the same ankle.

Initially, it would come on only when he walked fast or climbed stairs, but eventually, the pain became chronic. Whenever the pain seemed to get worse, he would visit his family physician, who would prescribe some pain killers for him. At one point, on his family physician's advice, Raman even began physiotherapy sessions.

However, he was not very regular with these, and eventually, he discontinued them as he thought they were not helping him in any way. One of Raman's friends had an older brother who was an orthopedic surgeon.

Raman and went to see him about five years ago. The doctor changed his pain medication and advised him about continuing his exercises. He assured him that with time his ankle would get better.

When Raman continued to have pain, he came to see us on the advice of a friend. By now, the pain was constant and he had developed a limp. Because of the bad ankle, for the past five years, Raman had been following a more or less sedentary lifestyle. He was presently overweight and in poor physical condition. He had gained about 15 kg in the last five years, which did nothing for his injured ankle.

On examination and imaging, we found that Raman had early arthritis in his right ankle. He also had chronic ligament injuries, which had not healed.

After informing him in detail about his diagnosis and the treatment options, we started his therapy. He underwent 5 to 6 sessions of Prolotherapy at Alleviate, and in about 3 months, Raman had remarkable improvement in his symptoms.

⁂

How did Raman's longstanding pain symptoms get better? How was he able to get back to his normal life? Raman not only returned to a pain-free life, but he also was physically in much better health. He lost weight and faced life with a positive outlook.

This change came about when he wholeheartedly followed the Alleviate Way of treatment. As you read through the chapters of this book, you will learn more about how we can help you manage your pain. It was surprising to us that Raman had not consulted a specialist for five years, but chose to live with his pain. This was because he was never given a diagnosis in his previous visits to various doctors. He became resigned to the pain. But when he was given a specific diagnosis and the treatment plan was spelled out, Raman was willing to give it his all for a better life. This involved a lot of lifestyle changes on his part, such as regular exercising and dieting. But the results were worth every effort on his part.

In conclusion, what I want to impress is this: Be sure of what ails you. Be prepared to do what it takes. It is not enough to just consult a competent physician or surgeon; you have to be prepared to do your part.

Whatever the method of therapy, be it surgery, regenerative treatments, or an interventional pain management procedure, you still have to be ready to fulfill your part of the bargain by committing to a regular exercise schedule, following healthy dietary habits, keeping track of your body weight, and adhering to positive lifestyle choices. In doing so you will reap the benefits for a long time.

'Toward a healthy pain-free life!'

2

DEGENERATIVE CASCADE OF ARTHRITIS

Maintenance is the magic word.

We are all familiar with the phrase, "running like a well-oiled machine." It basically refers to something that is running smoothly and efficiently and is functioning at its full potential. It could be a machine or it could be an organization as well! It goes without saying that such a machine is obviously under good maintenance.

The human body is connected or knit together with connective tissue elements like bones, tendons, and ligaments. The normal functioning of the body requires that all these structures work in tandem by getting their signals from the brain, which can be likened to the signal box of a machine. Appliances that we commonly use in our homes, such as washing machines, refrigerators, and automobiles seem to work perfectly well and quite efficiently in the initial years with very little maintenance. But as the years go by, if we have not looked after them the way we should have, we start to notice problems.

A neighbor, who bought a car of the same make as yours just a few months after you, appears to be enjoying absolutely trouble-free rides, whereas your mechanic has diagnosed a whole lot of repair works for your vehicle. So where is the difference?

Well, the neighbor has basically been taking good care of his car's health! He has made sure the vehicle was taken for servicing on schedule. He is a careful driver and his car has not been involved in any major accidents, except maybe for a couple of grazes. He makes sure to not push the car beyond its endurance for speed. On the other hand, you love speed and are constantly pushing your vehicle to its limit. You have been involved in two major accidents and the servicing has been haphazard at best. When you were visiting abroad, the car lay idle for nearly six months.

These are just two extreme scenarios with a vehicle owner. Anyone can be either of you or be somewhere in between when it comes to vehicle maintenance. It is quite clear that the longevity of the vehicle as well as its trouble-free performance is dependent on its maintenance. The same holds true for the human body. The various mobile parts of our locomotive system depend on good maintenance as well. The skeletal system in our body has numerous moving parts, and these are in use daily as long as we live.

Constant forces that act on the various attachments and articulations of the skeletal system can cause wear and tear at these points. For example, when bone rubs on bone due to degeneration of the intervening cartilage, arthritis ensues. Similarly, inflammation of a tendon caused by friction with a bone can cause tendonitis, such as Achilles tendonitis or Patellar tendonitis. Neglect and poor maintenance of the skeletal system can lead to a DEGENERATIVE CASCADE, and when the bones and joints are involved, arthritis is the result, with the involved bones touching (bone on bone) each other.

Arthritis Of The Knee Joint

The joint most commonly affected by arthritis is the knee joint.

The structure of the knee joint is quite complex and constitutes a number of structures that are mobile such as the lateral and medial menisci, cartilage, and the anterior and posterior cruciate ligaments.

We can understand that in a machine with multiple moving components, the dysfunction of a single part due to either a loose nut or bolt can lead to overcompensation by the other parts, thereby jeopardizing the structural integrity and the efficiency of the entire machine over a period of time. The same principle can be applied to the knee joint as well. When the natural cushioning that is present in the knee joint wears away, the support system is weakened.

The cartilage in the knee joint acts as the shock absorber of the joint, and when it experiences undue stress, it starts breaking down. This sets into motion the degenerative cascade and vicious circle of chronic pain.

It is important to remember that this process takes many years to progress, and is catalyzed by predisposing factors such as previous knee injuries, obesity, sedentary lifestyle, use of improper footwear, excessive use of stairs, constant walking over uneven terrain, and excessive squatting (commonly seen in rural Indians). These factors usually exist along with a casual or indifferent attitude toward the increasing disability.

Here are two examples of people suffering from knee pain set against the backdrop of life in the Indian Subcontinent

CASE STUDY 2

Mr. Mohan had grown up in Mumbai, India. He studied to become a computer engineer, and on completion of his education, he was employed by one of the major IT firms in Mumbai. Although Mohan had won many academic laurels in the course of his studies that he was quite proud of, he was not much of a sports person.

His physical activity had been limited to an occasional game of cricket on the weekends during his school and college days. When in his mid-thirties, Mohan was following a sedentary lifestyle, working in a high-pressure environment in a centrally airconditioned office. Compared to his weight during student days, he had now gained about 20 pounds. He was beginning to experience occasional stiffness and mild pain in his knee joints. Just as many of us would, Mohan too resorted to using over-the-counter pain medications, analgesic sprays, and oil preparations to obtain relief. He considered the pain to be a niggling matter that would probably run its course and disappear. All through his third decade, Mohan did not find it necessary to take any significant measures for the pain, which was an infrequent although unpleasant visitor. He was able to manage the incidents of pain with relative ease.

When he entered his forties, Mohan got a promotion in his work, which meant air travel about thrice a week. He found the work pressure to have increased about three times as well. For the past decade or so, Mohan had not undertaken any cardiovascular activity such as brisk walking, jogging, or cycling.

The knee pain too had changed in character. From being an infrequent visitor, the pain now was dictating certain areas of Mohan's life. He now avoided walking long distances or visiting hilly places. He was unable to play with his children as freely as his peers were doing, and he now found long flights to be a pain.

At this juncture, he decided to seek professional help and consulted three to four orthopedic surgeons. All of them unanimously gave him the same diagnosis—Arthritis! While one of the consultants was keen for him to undergo Total Knee Replacement (TKR), the others believed that as he was just 46 years old, it was too early for him to undergo surgery, and instead, he should focus on conservative measures such as diet, lifestyle modification, physical therapy, and regular exercise. Mohan too decided that surgery was not an option at such an early age, and he would be careful to follow all the lifestyle changes recommended by the experts.

Over the next few years, Mohan attempted to follow his resolutions, but he was not able to sustain his commitments for a meaningful period of time. He underwent three to four intermittent cycles of physiotherapy, and except for spurts of following a healthy diet and regular exercising, he found he was not able to keep his resolve. Mohan had always been a bright and jovial person, but by the time he reached his fifties, the limitations in his daily activities due to arthritis were taking a toll on his demeanor. He now avoided going out with his friends or any other activity that required prolonged periods of sitting or standing. He was not as cheerful as before, and his physical limitation was changing his outlook to pessimism in other walks of his life as well. Fast forward the scenario by a few years and we find Mr. Mohan, who is now 62 years old, lying on an operating table waiting to be anesthetized. He is praying to the Almighty that he might come out of surgery free from his long painful odyssey

CASE STUDY 3

Let us now look at Rita's story. Rita was born and brought up in a middle-class family in Mysore. She was an active child and always a great help to her mother whose days were usually swamped with household chores and the care of four children. Rita was pressured by her family to get married early, and at the tender age of 19, she gave in and married Mr. Basavaraju, a lawyer.

All of a sudden, the sprightly young girl with a glint in her eyes and great aspirations in her heart found herself in her mother's shoes. She was already in charge of a household! The little girl in Rita slowly vanished as she gradually got absorbed in running her home. In no time, Rita was the central focus of the Basavaraju family, and the entire household structure revolved around her.

Let us take a look at a day in Rita's life. Rita's day began with sweeping the entire house and then mopping the floor on her knees. She then cooked breakfast and lunch for her husband and children. During the course of the day, she climbed up and down three flights of stairs around three or four times, to dry clothes on the terrace and then fetch them when they had dried. She also sat cross-legged on the kitchen floor to do her various activities such as cleaning and sorting vegetables. Throughout the day she also attended to the needs of her recumbent father-in-law (recumbent, but no less demanding!). There was the preparation of dinner for the entire family and also running after her children to get things done.

This "homeathon" that she was running every day was certainly not kind or beneficial to her knees! Let us fast forward the scene by 4 decades. The years have definitely not been kind to Rita. She is now an insulin-dependent diabetic and has developed a heart condition as well.

Although her medical problems are well-controlled under the supervision of her family physician, who also happens to be her son's friend, the condition of her knees has crippled all the joy in her life. The mere sight of the flight of stairs that she so effortlessly ran up and down years ago makes her tremble at her knees.She is unable to sit cross-legged, and rising after sitting down for even 15 minutes makes her grimace in pain. Rita is blessed with two grandchildren who are quite a handful. Being around them brings out the whimsical child in her, but just a few quick steps chasing them is enough to bring on the knee pain, and the fun and games come to a grinding halt.

The years following her menopause have been even more painful. Her aunt has passed down five bottles of some oil to her, and she religiously massages this into her knees daily. She found some relief in the beginning, but now Rita knows deep down in her heart that the oil does not have even a placebo effect. The orthopedic surgeon has advised surgery, but Rita is petrified of going under the knife. One can see that she is dwindling away slowly, and unless corrective measures in terms of treatment, lifestyle, and exercise are taken, the knee pain will continue to play the devil with Rita's quality of life EVERY SINGLE DAY.

We may come across many such *Mohan*s and *Rita*s in real life. The stories may not match exactly, but bits and fragments of their history will be similar. As we learn from the above stories, the whole affair has taken not one or two days, but years to culminate in endless distress and pain. Arthritis of the joints is a degenerative process that begins in middle age and runs its course through two or three decades or even longer. A person has ample time and enough warning signs to sit up, take notice, and take control of the disease, but unfortunately very few pay heed to this impending disaster.

Let me at this juncture explain the casual attitude of people towards arthritis when compared to that towards other chronic diseases such as diabetes, hypertension, or chronic kidney disease. People have been aware for a long time that these diseases are associated with bodily dysfunction, organ failure, heart attack, uncontrolled infection, terminal damage to limbs, loss of sensation, permanent disability, and sometimes even death.

Arthritis is considered a condition with nagging pain in the joints, and in Indian society, people manage the pain for decades with groans, grimaces, oils, massages, and painkillers. Many patients with arthritis decide to wait till they reach a certain age before opting for TKR surgery, but it sometimes becomes an indefinite wait because of other comorbidities such as obesity, lack of strength in the quadriceps (thigh muscle), and poorly controlled diabetes.

In the initial stages of the disease, the diagnosis invariably slips under the radar, because people do not associate the condition with serious morbidity or mortality! This is the point where the biggest mistake is made.

The degenerative cascade of arthritis soon makes the sufferer a host to chronic pain, and eventually, the pain starts exercising its deleterious effects on the body and the mind. In the end, poor quality of life with limited ability is as less desirable as a permanent disability. If we understand and accept this concept, a lot can be done in the early stages to stem the progression of arthritis.

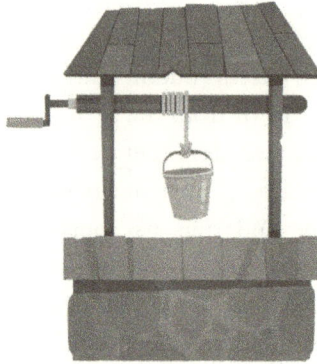

Human Knee Anatomy

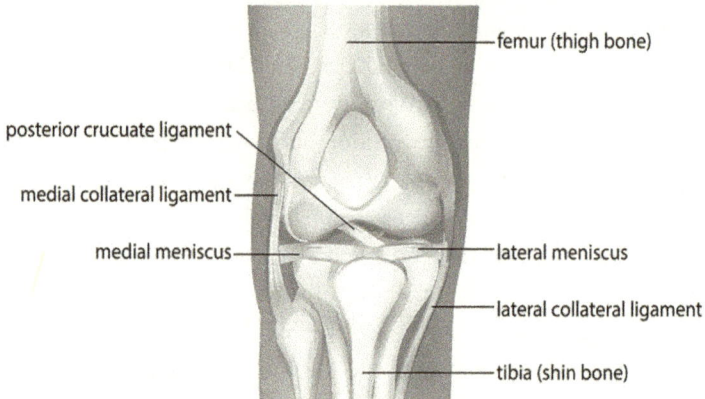

- femur (thigh bone)
- posterior crucuate ligament
- medial collateral ligament
- medial meniscus
- lateral meniscus
- lateral collateral ligament
- tibia (shin bone)

Breaking Down Arthritis

Let me explain the degenerative process of arthritis with this example. Imagine an old-fashioned well (let us call him Mr. Well!) in a busy town that has a rope and pulley mechanism and is used by a lot of people who draw water from it for domestic use. To make the analogy clearer, Mr. Well and the parts of his pulley system may be compared to the structure of the human knee joint.

The pulley represents the knee joint in the human body.

The nuts, bolts, and suspension can be compared to the soft tissue support in and around the knee joints, the primary ones being the menisci, cartilage, cruciate ligaments, and collateral ligaments. The rope used to pull up the bucket represents the quadriceps or thigh muscles and the bucket represents the leg below the knee joint.

When Mr. Well was inaugurated for use, it brought great joy to the poor people in the town. Since then, the pulley system of the well is probably one of the most used pieces of machinery in the town. Following streams of people lifting hundreds of buckets of water, and 16 to 18 hours of daily relentless labor, Mr. Well in three to four years, had started showing signs of fatigue. The initial damage was the loosening of the nuts and bolts that secured the pulley. If this had been spotted early and measures were taken, it would not have been difficult to rectify. But Mr. Well was public property and his duty was to serve!

Although there was plenty of gossip around him throughout the day concerning the affairs of the men and women in the town, Mr. Well did not so much as receive a caring glance from anyone.

Now the rope used to pull (quadriceps muscle) had weakened considerably, and this added undue pressure on the pulley (knee). The rope was at best changed once a year when it had frayed considerably and was close to giving way. So essentially, for most of the year, owing to the frayed and shredded condition of the rope, there was increased stress on the pulley. And no one had bothered to oil or lubricate the pulley mechanism since the day it was installed. This can be compared to the lubricant found in the knee joint, the synovial fluid.

Coming back to Mr. Well, lack of lubrication led to more than optimum friction across the pulley, which when repeated several times a day caused weakening of the structure. This explains exactly what happens in knee joint arthritis. Years of stress to the joints caused by excessive body weight, lax ligaments, previous injury in and around the joint, use of improper footwear, and a sedentary lifestyle are some of the causes that, acting individually or in tandem, can accelerate the degenerative process of arthritis.

What I wish to emphasize from this analogy is that had Mr. Well undergone regular maintenance, with timely repair work, oiling, and change of damaged components when required, he would have been able to serve his dependents for a very long time. In the same way, if people take good care of their knees by maintaining an ideal body weight, exercising regularly, and following a relatively healthy lifestyle, arthritis can be managed in a much better way.

The Alleviate Way:

Arthritis can be roughly divided into 4 stages ranging from mild to severe. The first two can be called the early stages and the last two, the late stages of arthritis. Patients who have early-stage arthritis with mild-to-moderate pain and stiffness can generally be considered candidates for regenerative therapy. At Alleviate, we treat most of our early arthritis patients with image-guided combination treatment of PLATELET RICH PLASMA, PROLOTHERAPY, and VISCOSUPPLEMENTATION. The procedure usually takes three to four sessions.

For those with severe arthritis, we recommend either Conventional Radiofrequency Treatment or COOLED Radiofrequency ablation of the genicular nerves for a longer duration of pain relief. The nerves around the knee joint are called the genicular nerves. For patients with moderate arthritis, we sometimes use both regenerative treatment as well as radiofrequency ablation for superior results. Steroids are generally used only in patients with rheumatoid arthritis.

Another modality of treatment used in knee joint arthritis is Intra-articular Ozone Infiltration. It is often used in conjunction with Radiofrequency treatment and Prolotherapy (PROLOZONE: Prolotherapy + Ozone). We try to address the problems faced by each and every patient by following a multidisciplinary approach.

We have on our team a Physical Therapist, a Clinical Nutritionist, a Clinical Psychologist, and a specialist in Preventive Medicine and Lifestyle Modification.

Irrespective of the stage of disease or the intervention that the patient is going for, they can avail the services of these specialists for wholesome and complete solutions tailored for them.

The key differentiating factor between a patient receiving great results and suboptimal results is their interest and involvement in whatever treatment option they are undergoing.

Finally, I would like to say that for those with intolerable knee pain and for those who are unable to bend their knee, if the other modalities of treatment are not of help and they are medically fit for surgery, they should consider TKR or Arthroplasty. This is a wonderful procedure when performed with the right indications.

But everyone must realize that TKR ought to be considered as a last resort or a terminal event, and there is much (exercise, nutrition, and lifestyle) each one can do as an individual over the period of two to three decades to not only delay the progression of arthritis but also keep ourselves fit for surgery should the need arise. It is significant that better candidates for surgery will also be able to uneventfully sail through the difficult postoperative rehabilitation period. Maintenance is the key to a trouble-free life, be it a machine or a human being.

3

BREAKING DOWN THE PARADIGM OF FIBROMYALGIA

It is not all in the mind!

Many a time a person complaining of diverse aches and pains may not really exhibit any obvious signs of a disease or cause externally. Sometimes they may not even have any focal point or relevant history to relate to the onset of pain. After a while, they may start to show a few behavioral changes and mood swings.

How do people deal with such a person? For a while, relatives and friends will be supportive, but eventually, they will be convinced that nothing is really wrong with the person and that he/she is imagining their symptoms of pain. It is all in your mind, will be the message.

Let us find out about Fibromyalgia, a condition that may not have really tangible signs, but which is definitely NOT ALL IN THE MIND!

Decoding Fibromyalgia

Fibromyalgia is a complex disorder that can present in multiple ways. It is a complex condition and not very well understood by either the common man or the health professionals. Why is that so?

The main symptoms of fibromyalgia are widespread pain and fatigue, which can actually be the presenting complaint for a whole lot of other disease conditions as well. And because it involves the nervous system, it can affect many different parts of the body. These factors make it very difficult for a doctor to diagnose fibromyalgia as the cause of a patient's aches and pains.

There is an old saying that you might have heard. The famous philosopher Henri Bergson said, *"The eyes see only what the mind is prepared to comprehend."* It can be paraphrased as "the eyes see and recognize only what the mind knows and understands." This is true in the case of fibromyalgia. Unless one is aware of this condition and the various ways it can present, it is very unlikely that a sufferer can be correctly diagnosed.

A physician will be able to diagnose any condition with ease and accuracy when it presents with a set of signs and symptoms peculiar to that particular condition. The other prerequisite for ease of diagnosis is a set of well-established investigative procedures that can confirm a diagnosis. In the absence of these factors, it is difficult to arrive at a diagnosis easily. The sad fact is that a lot of doctors are still quite unaware of the presentation, course, diagnosis, and management of fibromyalgia.

Fibromyalgia can actually be referred to as a syndrome rather than a single disease. Why do I say this? A collection of signs and symptoms that occur together is usually called a syndrome. Although the cardinal symptom of fibromyalgia is widespread body pain, the patient can also have a lot of other complaints concomitantly such as chronic tiredness, mood swings, and sleep disorders, to name a few. Owing to its complex presentation, the disease as such can affect the quality-of-life of the patient to a very great extent. That is why the early and accurate diagnosis of fibromyalgia is very essential.

In 1990, the American College of Rheumatology defined fibromyalgia and published their research findings, which now is the cornerstone for diagnosing fibromyalgia.

The condition is recognized to have a quartet of symptoms comprising **unexplained pain, easy fatiguability, frequent mood disturbances,** and **loss of function.**

Fibromyalgia is seen more commonly in women. The incidence in women has been found to be seven times more than that in men. The onset is most often in middle-age, but it can occur in the teens or in older age groups also.

Let us try to understand the story of fibromyalgia and what is behind its occurrence.

What Causes Fibromyalgia?

Over the years, a lot of theories have been put forward on the etiology of fibromyalgia, and while some have been discarded based on research, some theories have stood the test of time and are accepted either entirely or at least partly by the medical fraternity.

These are some of the pathologies that have been proposed in the development of fibromyalgia:

1. Soft tissue damage:

It was thought that injury or trauma that caused damage to soft tissues, such as muscles, tendons, or ligaments, might be the triggering factor for the onset of fibromyalgia. But this theory is not widely accepted as muscle biopsy studies have not shown any tissue damage that could be linked to the development of fibromyalgia.

2. Disturbances in Serotonin Epinephrine pathways:

Serotonin and epinephrine are two important neurotransmitters in our bodies. They play an inhibitory role in the transmission of pain signals from the different parts of the body to the brain.

That is, they help the brain in processing the stimuli received from other parts of the body. It has been found that in fibromyalgia, there are some disruptions in this pathway, and therefore the patients perceive increased pain in their muscles and tendons.

Stimuli such as mild pressure will be misinterpreted as pain when serotonin levels are decreased. This heightened perception of pain is known as "Central Sensitization." Basically, when you get hurt, something called a "flare" occurs and you feel the pain more.

3. Substance-P concentration:

Substance-P is an excitatory neurotransmitter. That means, it increases the perception of pain. It was initially thought that in fibromyalgia there was an increase in the concentration of Substance-P, and this was the reason for "central sensitization." But research thus far has failed to show a clear correlation between Substance-P levels and the degree of pain in patients.

4. Autoimmune causes:

It has been found that there are increased levels of cytokines such as Interleukin-2 in patients with fibromyalgia. Cytokines basically act as messengers between cells. They are involved in the regulation of inflammation in the body in response to infection or disease.

Some cytokines are pro-inflammatory, that is they increase the inflammatory response, while some are anti-inflammatory, with an opposite effect. Interleukin-2 is thought to be a pro-inflammatory cytokine, and therefore, increases the inflammatory response of the body. However, it is still unclear whether fibromyalgia causes the raised levels of Interleukin-2 or the other way around. On the contrary, many autoimmune conditions such as Inflammatory Bowel Disease and Rheumatoid Arthritis are found to be present concomitantly in fibromyalgia patients.

5. Sleep patterns:

Electroencephalogram (EEG) studies have shown that patients with fibromyalgia exhibit increased alpha brain wave activity and reduced delta brain wave activity in sleep. Brain waves are patterns of electrical activity that occur in the brain. There are 4 types of brain waves: Alpha, Beta, Theta, and Delta. Alpha waves are seen mainly in the awake state and Delta waves occur during sleep. The sleep EEG patterns in fibromyalgia patients suggest the role of sleep disturbances in its etiology. Reduced sleep may contribute to the low energy state and fatigue experienced in fibromyalgia, or pain may contribute to the sleep disturbances.

6. Hypothalamic-Pituitary axis involvement:

It is well known that hormones play an important role in the stress response of our body. The endocrine glands such as the hypothalamus and pituitary glands are involved in the production of these hormones. It has been suggested that some disturbances in the Hypothalamic-Pituitary Axis might lead to the development of fibromyalgia, although this has not been conclusively proven.

7. Changes in the Central and Peripheral Nervous System:

Some researchers have reported changes observed in the central and peripheral nervous system in people with fibromyalgia. Brain imaging studies have shown some changes in function and connections between different parts of the brain.

8. External Stress:

Other external stressful stimuli such as physical injury, emotional trauma, and physical or sexual abuse can play a role in triggering the symptoms of fibromyalgia.

Clinical Presentation

Although fibromyalgia is associated with a variety of symptoms, the most characteristic one is the presence of widespread pain. The pain is often accompanied by extreme fatigue, sleep dysfunction, and cognitive impairment. This means along with pain in different parts of their body, the person with fibromyalgia also experiences tiredness, inability to sleep well, and difficulty in remembering, performing daily activities, making decisions, and concentration. Let us learn about the 4 main (quartet) symptoms of fibromyalgia.

1. Pain

Patients with fibromyalgia usually give a history of bilateral pain. Pain is also present in axial structures like the cervical, thoracic, or lumbar areas of the spine or the chest wall. To make it easier, the American College of Rheumatology came out with the following diagnostic criteria in 1990:

- History of widespread pain for 3 months or more.
- Pain in at least 11/18 defined tender point sites on exertion of a force of 4 kg with the thumb.

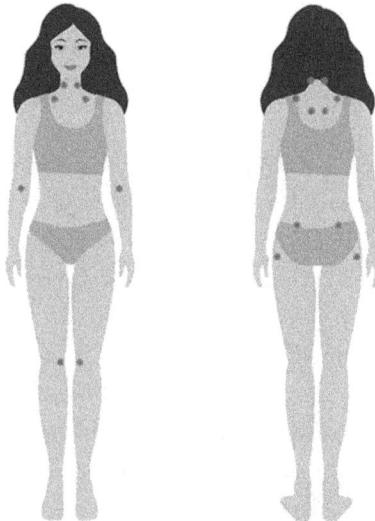

There are 18 tender point sites (nine pairs), which are situated symmetrically on both sides of the body. They basically cover the areas both above and below the waist: around the neck, chest, shoulders, hips, and knees.

1. Both sides of the back of the head: the occiput region
2. Both sides of the neck: near the lower cervical vertebrae, C5—C7
3. Top of each shoulder: midpoint or upper border of the trapezius muscle
4. Shoulder blades: around the origin of the supraspinatus muscle
5. Both sides of the upper chest: around the region of the second rib
6. Outside of each elbow: region of the lateral epicondyle
7. Both sides of the hips: upper and outer region of the buttocks
8. Buttocks: greater trochanter of the femur or thigh bone
9. Insides of the knees: close to the joint line medially
10. Fatigue

The patient suffering from fibromyalgia experiences chronic tiredness. This is characteristically termed 'daytime fatigue.' It can range from mild tiredness on some days to extreme exhaustion on certain other days. It is important to differentiate fatigue in fibromyalgia from another condition called Chronic Fatigue Syndrome. The basic difference is, in fibromyalgia, pain will be the dominant symptom, followed by tiredness, whereas, in Chronic Fatigue Syndrome, tiredness will be the main complaint with maybe slight body pain.

1. Sleep Disturbance

Patients with fibromyalgia experience what is called non-restorative sleep. That is, although they may sleep for the required number of hours, they will still be tired when they wake up.

Fibromyalgia patients have reported that they find it hard to fall asleep and also experience increased nighttime awakenings. Sleep recordings of the brain have shown that they tend to spend lesser time in deep sleep.

2. Cognitive Impairment

The various symptoms of fibromyalgia are probably interrelated, with one leading to the other. People with fibromyalgia experience difficulty in thinking, concentration, and decision-making. This condition is termed "fibro fog." Experts attribute this to the lack of sufficient deep sleep, which impairs brain functioning. Apart from the above-mentioned main quartet of symptoms, fibromyalgia patients may also present with the following complaints:

- **Joint Pain:**
  The tender points are very small areas and are usually near joints. But it is important to note that the joints themselves are not involved. Joint pain may be present when the patient is suffering from other concomitant diseases like Rheumatoid Arthritis.
- **Jaw Pain:**
  Patients with fibromyalgia may also have a condition called the temporomandibular joint (TMJ) syndrome. The TMJ is what connects the lower jaw (jaw bone) to the upper jaw (this is part of the skull). The various muscles and ligaments help in opening and closing the mouth. Pain or tenderness around the TMJ is referred to as TMJ syndrome. The most likely cause is trauma to the jaw bone.
- **Headaches:**
  It has been found that tension headaches and migraine are seen more frequently in those with fibromyalgia. Tension headaches are usually bilateral and do not worsen with activity. Migraine is typically one-sided and may worsen with activity.

- **Restless Legs Syndrome:**
  In this condition, people feel compelled to keep moving their legs. It is described as having an unpleasant sensation in the leg. The symptoms worsen at night. Restless legs syndrome is seen more often in patients with fibromyalgia.
- **Tingling and Numbness:**
  Changes in the brain that occur in fibromyalgia can make patients hypersensitive to pain stimuli. As a result, they may experience numbness and tingling in their limbs. While this may be present in the hands, in general, it is more commonly felt in the legs. This sensation is called paresthesia.
- **Anxiety and Depression:** Patients with fibromyalgia can present with disorders associated with anxiety and depression such as dysthymia, panic disorders, and phobias. Chronic pain, restriction in social activities, impact on profession, and inability to perform daily activities may be some of the factors that lead to depression in these patients. It is thought that pain and depression probably aggravate each other during the course of fibromyalgia.

Diagnosis

The following are the important points to be noted in the diagnosis of FM:

- History of pain for more than 3 months
- Generalized pain in 4/5 major body regions
    - (a) Left upper region (shoulder, arm, jaw)
    - (b) Right upper region (shoulder, arm, jaw)
    - (c) Left lower region (hip, buttock, leg)
    - (d) Right lower region (hip, buttock, leg)
    - (e) Axial region (neck, back, chest, abdomen)

1. **Exclusion of other conditions through tests and imaging**

The diagnosis of FM can be called a diagnosis of exclusion. This is due to the fact that there is no single test or investigation that can confirm the diagnosis of FM. Moreover, almost all the symptoms experienced by patients with FM can be present in numerous other medical conditions as well.

To facilitate the diagnosis of FM, the American College of Rheumatology has framed some diagnostic criteria. These help in the preliminary diagnosis of FM and also in assessing the severity of the symptoms experienced by the patients. Scores are given on the Widespread Pain Index and the Symptom Severity Scale.

Another assessment method is the **Fibromyalgia Impact Questionnaire**. This questionnaire carries 20 questions that help to quantify the impact of the disease on patients. It helps in assessing the components of health that are most affected by FM. It is self-administered and can be completed in 5 minutes. It is simple to use and self-explanatory. You can find the questionnaire online.[1]

The scoring on this questionnaire will range from 0 to 100, and most fibromyalgia patients will obtain a score above 50. A score greater than 70 can indicate that the patient is severely affected.

Another questionnaire that can be used is the **Fibromyalgia Survey Questionnaire**. This is mainly used in research and survey settings where detailed tender point examination and evaluation of the number of pain sites and symptom severity may be difficult. This is a simpler questionnaire for the patients to answer. This is also found online.

In addition to administering the questionnaire, the patient must also be thoroughly checked for the presence of other conditions that can cause similar symptoms. Conditions such as hypothyroidism, rheumatoid arthritis, systemic lupus erythematosus (SLE), and other inflammatory states must be investigated and ruled out.

---

[1]https://www.physio-pedia.com/Fibromyalgia_Impact_Questionnaire_(FIQ)

Chronic conditions such as TMJ disease and chronic fatigue syndrome must also be ruled out. Mrs. Latha Seshadri, a college professor, found her life turned upside down as a result of some undiagnosed problem. She tried many remedies, but no one could help her. Let us find out more about her

CASE STUDY 4

Mrs. Latha Seshadri, a 47-year-old lady from Mumbai, came to us with a history of long-standing pain and feeling of tiredness. She was a college professor but had not been working for the past two years owing to her physical ailments. Latha had always been a very active person, who took advantage of every opportunity that came her way. Right from her school days, she was involved in multiple activities apart from her studies. She was keenly interested in sports and had represented her school in a number of athletic events. She continued to be a vivacious person all through her college life as well. On completion of her studies, her parents fixed her marriage to Mr. Seshadri, a telecom officer working in Mumbai.

Soon Latha settled into her married life in Mumbai. She joined a reputed college as a junior lecturer and as was her usual style, dived wholeheartedly into academic life. Her students loved her and she was a positive influence on all who came across her. Her first son was born when she was 26 years old, and in a couple of years, she gave birth to a girl.

Latha managed her home and professional life equally, and all her colleagues marveled at her abilities. She was always on the go, seeing to her children and husband's needs, but at the same time ensuring that her students were not neglected. The family lived in telecom quarters provided for her husband, and Latha had a daily long commute to her college by local train. In the initial years, she did not find the commute difficult or tiresome, and life rolled along.

After a few years, Latha started feeling increasingly tired on returning home from work. She found she was not able to devote the same energy and enthusiasm to her home duties as before. She started experiencing pain in different parts of her body. It was generalized pain that was initially present on and off. She attributed this to standing for long hours on the local trains.

As she generally had a positive nature, she did not worry too much about the body pain and tiredness and thought of ways to overcome them. Her husband arranged a driver to take her to college and back every day. Latha felt she had neglected to exercise regularly and maintain her body in the years following childbirth. She started walking daily to improve her physical fitness.

Although her symptoms seemed to get better initially, they recurred with more intensity. Latha now had to take over-the-counter pain killers, but that did not seem to help much. She felt tired most of the time She was not sleeping well and did not have any interest in her home. Whatever energy she had was devoted to her profession.

By the time Latha was in her forties, her pain symptoms had increased to the level that her quality of life had markedly deteriorated. She was unable to work for almost 15 days in a month. She was depressed and moody and avoided all social contact. She tried numerous home remedies such as oil massages and application of local balms on the advice of her friends and relatives to no avail. She came to see us on the recommendation of a colleague. When we saw her, she was markedly depressed, unable to perform her daily activities, and in considerable pain. She was also confused about her condition, as none of the physicians she had consulted thus far had been able to pinpoint a diagnosis.

Our team assessed her, by first obtaining a comprehensive medical history. This was followed by a complete physical examination. All relevant investigations and tests to rule out other possible conditions were carried out. Apart from being slightly overweight and having mild hypertension, she did not have any other medical conditions.

A diagnosis of fibromyalgia was made based on these factors, and a multidisciplinary approach was taken to manage her symptoms. Just the knowledge that her symptoms were not imaginary, but instead presented a disease condition, helped improve her outlook. We gave her information about fibromyalgia and the various treatment modalities that are available for managing the condition. She was treated with trigger point injections and physiotherapy. She was taught various self-help tips that she can follow easily on her own to manage her symptoms. Our lifestyle consultant helped her with suggestions to make appropriate changes in her daily routine to reduce her symptoms. She and her family members were given counseling and informed about the available resources. She showed remarkable improvement in her condition following two weeks of therapy. She left for Mumbai feeling more in control of her life and her condition. The diagnosis of her disease and the assurance of help made all the difference.

As mentioned earlier, fibromyalgia can be the primary disease or it can coexist with other chronic diseases. In fact, these other chronic conditions may have a role in the etiopathogenesis of fibromyalgia in a patient. This is what happened with Radhika. Although she was diagnosed with her primary condition fairly soon and started appropriate therapy, something was missed. Let's find out.

CASE STUDY 5

Radhika was a 35-year-old IT professional who was referred to us by her doctor. She had been diagnosed with Inflammatory Bowel Disease (IBD) about three years before. IBD is an autoimmune condition, where the patient develops severe inflammation in different parts of the intestine. They can present with various symptoms such as diarrhea, tiredness, abdominal pain and cramping, fatigue, and decreased appetite.

She was treated with anti-inflammatory medicines, and when necessary, steroids to control 'flare-ups' of the disease. The disease was initially under control and Radhika was able to continue her normal life. About one year later, she started experiencing a lot of body pain and tiredness. The condition was thought to be a flare-up of IBD and treated accordingly. Symptoms of a flare-up can vary from person to person, but they usually present with joint pain, fatigue, lack of appetite, etc.

Flare-ups usually last for days or weeks, and then the patient goes into remission again. However, in Radhika's case, the symptoms were not getting better. She was increasingly tired and could not attend work on many days. She did not sleep well at night and seemed to be disoriented in the daytime. She was unable to perform her daily household work and was depressed and anxious.

On suggestion from her colleagues and friends, she even joined a meditation course. Nothing seemed to help her. Finally, her brother took her to a specialist, who after going through her records carefully sent her to us. After assessing her properly, we were able to diagnose the presence of concomitant fibromyalgia. This had been undetected for more than a year. The stress from the IBD might have been the initial trigger for the condition. Again, we took a multi-disciplinary approach to manage her symptoms. She was given trigger-point injections and joint injections for the pain. She underwent physiotherapy and counseling. She was taught exercises that she could do easily along with other self-help tips to manage her symptoms. Our Life-Style Consultant was able to advise on aspects of proper nutrition, fitness, etc. Reassuring the patient has a very positive effect. To know that there is help and we are there for moral support gives hope to these patients and they feel that they can get better.

Investigations

The following blood tests can help in identifying the presence of other inflammatory conditions and autoimmune diseases that need to be ruled out in the patient.

- Complete blood cell count (CBC): The CBC evaluates all the cells circulating in the blood. For instance, in an infection, the total WBC count may increase. In certain vitamin deficiencies, the RBCs may show abnormal shapes. Particular white blood cells may show an increase in inflammatory conditions.
- Erythrocyte sedimentation rate (ESR): This test basically determines how quickly the blood cells settle in the bottom of a test tube following agitation. An increased rate can indicate inflammatory conditions like SLE or Rheumatoid arthritis
- Muscle enzyme levels: Certain muscle enzymes may be elevated in other conditions that cause pain in muscles. For example, muscle injury or muscular dystrophy.
- Thyroid Function Tests: Thyroid hormone levels can point to a disorder of the thyroid gland.
- Rheumatoid factor: This test can show high levels in autoimmune conditions, mainly, rheumatoid arthritis.
- Antinuclear antibodies (ANA): A positive ANA test indicates the presence of an autoimmune disease.
- Vitamin D levels: Low levels indicate Vitamin D deficiency, where patients can present with chronic fatigue and persistent headache.

Treatment

The goal in the treatment of fibromyalgia should be to reduce pain, improve sleep, and relieve other associated conditions like fatigue, depression, and impaired cognition. No single therapy is effective in combating all the symptoms. Both medications and self-care strategies have been found effective in relieving symptoms of fibromyalgia. Patients have to try and decide on the combination that best works for them. The treatment modalities on offer for fibromyalgia patients may be classified broadly as

(A) Pharmacological and (B) Non-pharmacological therapy.

(a) Pharmacological Treatment:

I. Antidepressants:

These are medicines that are commonly prescribed for patients with depression. Tricyclic antidepressant Amitriptyline in low doses ranging from 25 to 50 mg/day has been used in the treatment of fibromyalgia. It acts by increasing the serotonin levels in the body. It also has a sedative effect.

In some patients, it is known to improve symptoms of pain, fatigue, sleep disturbance, and depression. However, it must be taken with careful monitoring as patients may have side effects like weight gain or develop tolerance, requiring increasingly higher doses.

Serotonin Noradrenaline Reuptake Inhibitors (SNRIs) are another class of antidepressants that are being used in treating fibromyalgia. They are thought to help by increasing the serotonin and norepinephrine levels in the body, leading to better brain function, such as increased alertness, good mood, and retrieval of memory. Duloxetine is an SNRI that has been recommended for use in the dose of 60 mg/day. It is known to improve symptoms of fibromyalgia and reduce pain in some patients.

Another SNRI that is recommended is Milnacipran. It is given in the dose of 100 mg/day in divided doses. Studies have reported that this drug was found to improve fibromyalgia symptoms in only a small group of patients.

II. Anti-epileptic drugs:

Drugs used for seizure disorders such as Pregabalin and Gabapentin have been advocated for use in fibromyalgia patients. They act by decreasing the serum levels of Substance P, which is increased in fibromyalgia. They help by promoting sleep, decreasing anxiety levels, and modulating the pain.

The maximum recommended dose of Pregabalin is 100 mg thrice a day. Gabapentin may be prescribed in higher doses. These drugs must be taken only under the guidance of the treating physician.

III. Anti-inflammatory drugs:

Over-the-counter pain killers like Paracetamol and Ibuprofen are not effective in the management of fibromyalgia symptoms.

Tramadol is a weak Serotonin-Norepinephrine antagonist and has been found to reduce pain. Pramipexole, which is a drug used in the treatment of Parkinsonism, has been found to relieve fibromyalgia pain in some cases. Memantine is usually used in the treatment of Alzheimer's disease. It has been recommended for use in the treatment of fibromyalgia. It is thought to reduce pain symptoms by decreasing glutamate levels in the body.

Narcotic analgesics are generally contraindicated in the management of fibromyalgia because of their side effects and the development of dependence and tolerance of the drug following long-term use.

IV. Intravenous Infusions:

(i) **Myer's Cocktail:** A cocktail has been found effective in managing fibromyalgia symptoms. This is interesting news indeed! But this is not as you might imagine a fruity drink, but a concentrated dose of vitamins and minerals that is given intravenously once a week. Myer's cocktail is a formulation first proposed by Dr. John Myers, M.D., a physician from Baltimore, USA.

He experimented with a mix of vitamins and minerals such as the B-complex vitamins, vitamin C, magnesium, and calcium. Many patients and physicians have reported that this cocktail infusion has helped to significantly reduce pain and fatigue.

The following constitute Myer's Cocktail:

- 5 ml magnesium chloride hexahydrate (20%)
- 3 ml calcium gluconate (10%)
- 1 ml hydroxocobalamin (1000 μ/ml)
- 1 ml pyridoxine hydrochloride (100 mg/ml)
- 1 ml dexapanthenol (250 mg/ml)
- 1 ml B-complex 100 containing

a) 100 mg thiamine HCl, 2 mg riboflavin, 2 mg pyridoxine HCl, 2 mg panthenol
b) 100 mg niacinamide, 2% benxyl alcohol

- 5 ml Vitamin C (500 mg/ml)
- 20 ml sterile water

The whole infusion amounts to 37 ml and is colored a bright yellow. The exact mechanism of action is not very clear, but it is thought that magnesium and calcium may play a role in the dilatation of blood vessels, which in turn helps in increasing muscle oxygen supply. This may be beneficial in chronic fatigue. It is also believed that infusing vitamins and minerals directly into the bloodstream increases their bioavailability to the cells. The infusion is given through an intravenous drip and the entire procedure may take 30 to 45 minutes. There are no serious side effects that have been reported, except for a fall in blood pressure as magnesium can dilate the blood vessels. The patient is monitored throughout, and in case of falling blood pressure, the rate of infusion is slowed down.

(ii) **Lidocaine Infusions:** There are reports in recent times that intravenous infusion with Lidocaine, a local anesthetic, has been beneficial in improving pain as well as quality-of-life in patients with fibromyalgia. It is not recommended for use in people who have ECG abnormalities or electrolyte imbalance. Patients who have not improved with other traditional remedies can definitely try this treatment.

(iii) **Ketamine Infusions:** Ketamine is again an anesthetic drug that acts by causing dissociative anesthesia. That is, it can induce a trance-like state and a sense of disconnection. It is used by surgeons for short procedures or as a pre-anesthetic for general anesthesia. It is also an analgesic, and in low doses, it can relieve pain. Ketamine is thought to relieve pain in fibromyalgia patients by blocking the NMDA receptors. This causes decreased perception of pain. Ketamine should be used only under the supervision of a medical practitioner.

(b) Non-pharmacological Therapy

We have seen that fibromyalgia is a very challenging chronic pain condition and there is no single treatment for relieving the symptoms. Apart from the various medicines that were discussed in the previous section, there is much that patients can do to decrease their symptoms. Patient self-care is vital for improving symptoms and daily function. It cannot be stressed enough that a multidisciplinary approach is the key to managing symptoms and improving the quality of life in fibromyalgia. So, what are the different ways to approach the condition?

- Patient Education: Encourage the patient with fibromyalgia to read and learn about their condition. Patients should also be taught how they can improve their sleep patterns, concentration, etc.
- Regular Exercise: Exercise plays a role in restoring the body's neurochemical balance by increasing the secretion of feel-good neurotransmitters, leading to a positive mental state. Regular exercising allows patients to have some control over the disease and the amount of pain they feel.
- Cognitive Therapy: Counselors can help the patients to believe in themselves and give them strategies for dealing with stressful situations.

- Relaxation Techniques: Learning to reduce the tension in muscles called progressive muscle relaxation is helpful in some patients. Meditation and practicing yoga have also helped fibromyalgia patients. Each one has to choose what best suits them.
- Stress Management: Patients are taught to pace themselves. They are taught how to avoid overexertion and emotional stress. Deep breathing exercise routines have been helpful in some patients.

Apart from these, activities such as high-intensity aerobic exercises and aqua therapy have helped reduce symptoms in a few patients, but these activities may not be suitable for all. As we have seen, not only a multidisciplinary approach is necessary for managing this disease, patients also need a lot of emotional support from their families and therapists.

Living With Fibromyalgia

After you or someone close to you has been diagnosed with fibromyalgia, what can you do?

Here are some important points to remember:

- It is NOT a psychological condition!
- You are NOT being lazy!
- It is NOT whining or malingering!

Convey to the patient that their symptoms are real and there is help for it. If you are the patient, follow the advice of the doctors and therapists who are involved in your care, as they try to frame the best-suited remedies for you

What can you do from your side?

I have provided some basic SELF-CARE STEPS that you can follow and that will help you have control over your life.

1. Time to relax daily: Schedule a set time to relax, meditate, or do deep breathing exercises daily.

2. Set regular sleep pattern: Practice going to bed at the same time daily. Avoid daytime napping, which might disrupt your night sleep. Those who smoke should try to cut down or stop the habit altogether as nicotine is a stimulant and can disrupt sleep. Excessive coffee drinking can also be disruptive to your sleep as caffeine is a stimulant as well.

3. Exercise daily: Start with small attempts at gentle exercises. As your medications begin to work and pain decreases, you can slowly increase your exercise routine. Start Low and Go Slow. Take small walks and restart activities that you had stopped due to the pain.

4. Daily routine: Create a routine that you are comfortable with. You need not do everything all at once. Remember the saying—Rome was not built in a day! Read about your disease. Experiment and decide what best suits you. Develop a positive attitude! Keep your focus on what will make you better.

As we saw in the first case study, fibromyalgia turned Latha, an ambitious hardworking person, into someone who was constantly tired and disinterested, unable to perform even the basic daily activities. Or, in the case of Radhika, undiagnosed fibromyalgia made life with an existing chronic disease greatly unbearable. In ALLEVIATE, we provide a complete multidisciplinary approach to treating fibromyalgia. Our doctors, physiotherapists, psychologists, nutritionists, and lifestyle consultants work as a team to identify and provide the best-suited modalities of treatment for each individual patient. More than anything, we are there to reassure every patient that we are there to help and support them through their journey.

4

CHRONIC PAIN GENERATORS
IN THE SPINE

All back pain is not disc pain!

Ever since mankind evolved to stand erect on its hind feet, considerable stress has been placed on the spine or what is known as the backbone. All of us have experienced back pain at some point in our lives, or we are acquainted with someone, either a family member or a friend, who has experienced back pain or pain in the lumbar region. People commonly associate back pain with vertebral disc involvement as that is a widely known condition, but there can be numerous other causes for back pain as well.

When the pain lasts for only a couple of days before resolving, we are able to deal with it. But when the pain is constant or longstanding, it seriously impacts the quality of life of the affected person. Let us study the structure of the spine and its role in maintaining posture and giving support. This will help you to better understand the reasons why back pain occurs.

Structure Of The Spine

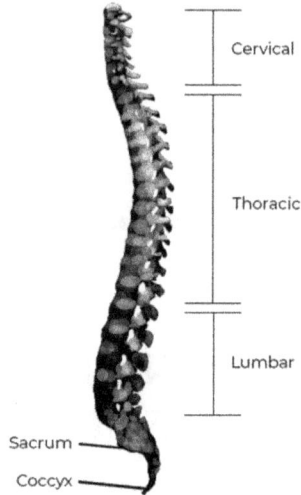

Human Vertebrae Anatomy

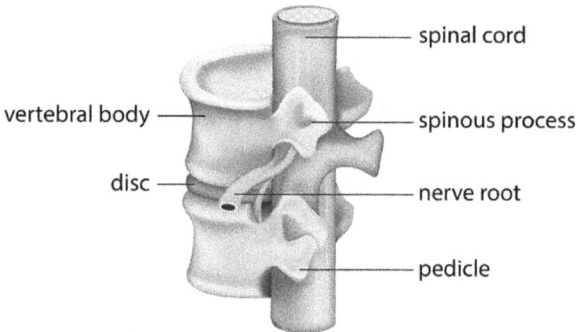

The spinal column in man is made up of 33 vertebral bones that are placed one on top of the other. The first set of 7 vertebrae is known as the cervical spine. This is followed by the thoracic spine, which consists of 12 vertebrae. Next comes the lumbar spine with 5 vertebrae, followed by the sacrum, which has 5 fused vertebrae, and the coccyx with 4 fused vertebrae.

Only the upper 24 vertebral bones are mobile and have the intervertebral disc between them. The bones in the sacrum and coccyx are fused. This structure of the spine can be compared to that of a multistorey building. The lower lumbar vertebrae can be compared to the basement or foundation of the building and they take up most of the strain.

We can understand that structural damage to any floor of a building can in turn cause increased pressure on the other floors, which in turn can damage the other floors and also compromise the structural integrity of the building.

The lower lumbar vertebrae can be compared to the basement of the building, which would bear maximum strain in case of damage to any of the upper floors. This is the reason why people commonly suffer from low back pain. Any pathology in the upper vertebral bones will eventually end up affecting the lower lumbar vertebrae.

Chronic Low Back Pain

A person is said to suffer from chronic low back pain (CLBP) if he/she presents with pain in the lower back for at least three months. CLBP is reported to be a leading cause of disability in the world, giving rise to considerable economic problems in the population and requiring state welfare measures. The prevalence of CLBP in adults is said to have more than doubled in the last decade.

It continues to increase drastically in the older population, significantly impacting their day-to-day functioning as well as their occupational activities.

CLBP can arise as a result of various conditions affecting not only the vertebral bones per se, but also the joints, muscles, tendons, and ligaments associated with the lumbar spine.

Psychological causes such as stress, depression, and anxiety are also said to play a role in the occurrence of CLBP. Owing to the complex web of causes behind CLBP, the evaluation and diagnosis of this condition can be challenging to the physician and requires careful clinical decision making.

Pain Generators

Pain in the lumbar spine can originate from the following structures (pain generators):

1. Intervertebral disc (Discogenic pain)

This is one of the commonest types of low back pain. It arises when the intervertebral disc gets damaged following trauma or other degenerative causes like aging. The intervertebral disc is a fibrocartilaginous cushion present between the vertebrae in the spinal column. It is composed of three main parts: the outer annulus fibrosis, the inner nucleus pulposus, and the cartilaginous endplates. Following trauma or aging, the disc can undergo desiccation, dehydration, etc. In these conditions, the nucleus pulposus migrates out through defects in the annulus and this can result in derangement in the arrangement of nerve fibers and blood vessels, leading to high levels of chemical mediators of inflammation and resulting in classical discogenic pain.

2. Nerve roots or ganglion (Radicular pain)

Radicular pain occurs due to compression of the nerve roots. It usually radiates from the hips and buttocks and shoots down through the legs. The condition is commonly known as sciatica. Here ectopic nerve discharges from the nerve roots or the dorsal ganglia are the cause of pain. It is commonly caused by chemical inflammation following disc herniation. Diagnosis calls for correlation between clinical and MRI findings.

3. Spinal cord (pain caused by spinal stenosis)

Certain conditions such as herniation of the vertebral disc, thickening of the ligaments, overgrowth of the articular processes, and scar tissue resulting from previous surgical procedures can cause progressive narrowing of the central canal and the lateral recess of the spinal cord. This leads to compression of the spinal cord and the neurovascular structures that traverse it. Patients typically present with neurogenic claudication, altered sensation, and occasional motor weakness.

Neurogenic claudication means the patient has intermittent leg pain resulting from compression of the nerves in the spinal cord. The patient might experience sensations of tingling and pain, which are referred to as altered sensations. The pain will increase on prolonged standing or extension of the spine, and the patient will feel better when they bend forward or stoop.

4. Facet Joints

These are the plain joints that are present between the articular processes of the vertebrae. The facet joints help connect two adjacent vertebrae. They are weight-bearing joints and can undergo some degenerative changes resulting in an arthritis-like condition known as facet joint syndrome. This condition can be caused by injuries, repetitive movements, poor posture, obesity, etc.

Here, the patients typically experience low back pain around the midline, and the pain usually does not radiate beyond the buttocks.

It has been reported that up to 30 percent of patients with CLBP may be suffering from facet joint involvement. The painful stimuli (nociception) in facet joint involvement usually originates from the synovial membrane, hyaline cartilage, bone, or fibrous capsule of the facet joint.

5. Sacroiliac Joint

This joint connects the spine to the pelvic bone or the hip bone. There are two sacroiliac (SI) joints in the body, one on either side. This joint plays a major role in stability and therefore allows only minimal movement. In SI joint disease, the pain is typically in the region of the posterior superior iliac spine.

It may radiate down, but unlike sciatica pain, it will not shoot down the legs. The pain may be aggravated by disturbances in sleeping and sitting postures, or sitting for too long. Pain in the SI joint can originate from arthritic bony surfaces, capsular distension, inflammation of the fascial or tendinous portions of the SI ligaments, or hypermobility of the joint due to sustained exposure to shear forces.

6. Piriformis Muscle

The piriformis muscle can go into spasm and compress the sciatic nerve. The resulting irritation of the sciatic nerve leads to the development of sciatica-like symptoms, with pain more in the buttock region. This is known as the piriformis syndrome.

There are a few other pain generators that can cause CLBP:

- Thickening and inflammation of ligaments: anterior longitudinal ligament (ALL), posterior longitudinal ligament (PLL), and interspinous ligaments
- Fractures
- Trigger points or myofascial pain

We have seen all the structures (generators) in the spine that can cause back pain. Now let us look into specific conditions that lead to CLBP and the steps involved in making a diagnosis.

When a patient presents to a physician with a complaint, the physician studies the symptoms (complaints of the patient) and the signs (elicited by the physician during examination). From this, the physician now has a set of working or probable diagnoses, which are called differential diagnoses.

Next, the physician takes the help of investigative procedures such as blood tests and imaging techniques to confirm the exact diagnosis.

Conditions Causing Chronic Low Back Pain

As we have seen, there are many structures in the back that can give rise to pain apart from the intervertebral disc. Below are some of the conditions that can give rise to CLBP.

Sacroiliac Joint Involvement

Anatomy:

The sacroiliac (SI) joint is the largest axial joint in the body, with an average surface area of 17.5 cm². It connects the spine to the pelvis. It basically helps in transferring stress forces from the spine to the hip bone and the legs. The adult SI joint displays a wide variability with regard to size, shape, and surface contour. There may be great disparity seen in these parameters between the two SI joints in the same individual. The SI joint is most often described as a large, auricular-shaped, diarthrodial synovial joint. In reality, only the anterior third of the interface between the sacrum and ilium is a true synovial joint; the rest of the joint comprises an intricate set of ligamentous connections.

The main function of this ligamentous system is to limit motion in all planes of movement. In women, the ligaments are weaker, thereby allowing increased mobility during normal childbirth or parturition. These senescent changes accelerate during the third and fourth decades of life and are manifested by surface irregularities, crevice formation, fibrillation, and clumping of chondrocytes. The iliac surface of the joint tends to get affected first and the degenerative changes on the sacral side generally lag by 10 to 20 years.

Innervation:

The innervation of the SI joint remains a subject of much debate. The innervation pattern can vary among different individuals.

Some experts say that the lateral branches of the L4–S3 dorsal rami provide most of the innervation to the posterior SI joint. Other investigators claim that L3 and S4 also contribute to the posterior nerve supply. The innervation of the anterior joint is similarly ambiguous.

Early 20th-century German literature asserts the anterior SI joint is supplied by the obturator nerve, superior gluteal nerve, and the lumbosacral trunk. Based on more recent publications, the anterior joint is thought to be innervated by either L2–S2 or L4–S2 dorsal rami. Function and Biomechanics: The SI joints are designed primarily for the stability of the body in the standing position. The functions of this joint include the transmission and dissipation of truncal loads to the lower extremities, limiting X-axis rotation, and facilitating childbirth.

When compared to the lumbar spine, the SI joints can withstand a medially directed force 6 times greater, but only half the torsion and 1/20th of the axial compression load. These last 2 motions may preferentially strain and injure the weaker anterior joint capsule.

Prevalence:

ALMOST 30 PERCENT OF LOW BACK PAIN ORIGINATES FROM THE SACROILIAC JOINT.

Mechanism of Injury: The mechanism of SI joint injury has previously been described as a combination of axial loading and abrupt rotation. This can happen if the person performs a twisting motion while carrying a heavy object. On an anatomic level, pathologic changes affecting many different SI joint structures can lead to nociception. These include capsular or synovial disruption, inflammation of the SI ligaments, arthritic changes in the bony surface of the joint, etc.

Causes of SI Joint Pain: The causes of SI joint pain can be attributed to two events: (a) joint disruption or (b) joint degeneration.

Joint disruptions occur abruptly usually following trauma. Joint degenerations, on the other hand, develop over a period of time.

(a) SI joint disruption:

- Motor vehicle accident
- Fall on the buttock
- Sudden lifting/twisting movements
- Natural childbirth

(b) SI joint degeneration:

- Previous fusion surgery of the spine
- Stress caused by leg length difference
- Osteoarthritis
- Infection of SI joint
- Paget's disease
- Rheumatoid arthritis

Symptoms:

1. Low back pain centered around the posterior aspect of the SI joint.
2. The pain may be referred to the buttocks and thighs, but does not extend below the knee.
3. Inability to sit for too long in the same position.
4. Activities such as sitting down, lying on the side of the pain, or climbing stairs can bring on the pain.

Pain in SI joint disease may be on one side or both sides. The pain may also be referred over a wide zone covering areas such as the lumbar spine, abdomen groin, thigh, foot, and ankle.

Treatment: The treatment of SI joint pain is known to be one of the most challenging problems confronting pain physicians. This is evident from the plethora of therapies that have been advocated for this disorder. Broadly, the treatment can be classified into 2 categories:

53

(a) therapy aimed at correcting the underlining pathology and (b) therapy aimed at alleviating symptoms. For complete healing to take place, it is very important to identify and treat other underlying psychosocial issues as well. This is best accomplished by following a multidisciplinary approach.

(1) Conservative Management: The non-interventional management of SI joint pain should ideally address the underlining pathology. In patients with true or apparent leg length discrepancy, shoe inserts may be used to help equally distribute the load borne by the SI joints. Leg length discrepancies are frequently found in asymptomatic individuals, and many patients have learned to compensate for this difference by altering their gait or posture; therefore, most experts recommend caution in using inserts and suggest the initial correction of only half the incongruity. In patients having SI joint pain resulting from altered gait mechanics and spine malalignment, physical therapy, and osteopathic or chiropractic manipulation have been reported to reduce pain and improve mobility. However, there are no prospective, controlled studies supporting these modalities. Nonsurgical stabilization programs have also been advocated for the management of SI joint pain; for example, the application of pelvic belts that reduce the sagittal rotation of incompetent SI joints in pregnant women.

(2) Intra-articular Injections: Intra-articular injections with a steroid preparation and/or a local anesthetic (LA) often help both in the diagnosis as well as treatment of SI joint disease. It has been reported in multiple studies that radiologically guided SI joint injections provided good-to-excellent pain relief lasting from 6 months to 1 year in most but not all cases.

(3) Proliferative therapy: Proliferative therapy (prolotherapy) has been advocated as a treatment for nonspecific LBP and SI joint pain. This involves the injection of certain natural substances such as dextrose, glycerin, or phenol. This is said to promote the growth of connective tissue, thereby strengthening and repairing weakened or damaged tendons and ligaments. The rationale behind the use of "prolotherapy" is that the ligaments and other soft tissue structures play a major role in the development of LBP. Thus, the injection of a drug promoting fibroblast hyperplasia should theoretically increase the strength and reduce sensitization of these structures.

(4) Radiofrequency Denervation Procedures: Radiofrequency (RF) denervation procedures have been used by several investigators to provide prolonged pain relief to patients suffering from SI joint pain. The techniques used have ranged from denervating the nerves supplying the SI joint to creating lesions in the joint itself, with one study reporting the use of a combination of the two. Targeting the nerve supply resulted in a higher success rate of pain relief than that seen with interventions that focused on the joint itself, with approximately two-thirds of the patients reporting significant pain relief. The major drawback to percutaneous RF denervation procedures is that they do not alleviate pain emanating from the ventral SI joint.

Mrs. Murthy's journey to a correct diagnosis for her back pain will help you understand how easily the right cause can be missed, leading to unnecessary suffering and pain.

CASE STUDY 6

Mrs. Murthy is an elderly lady who presented to our clinic with longstanding back pain. She had been suffering from this pain since her early forties. In the initial days, she tried a lot of home remedies, and on the advice of her neighbors and well-wishers, she also tried out various local treatments like applying some oils and massaging the back. Eventually, she resorted to taking painkillers, but she did not experience permanent relief from the pain. She was told that disc surgery would cure her pain and accordingly she underwent fusion surgery of the spine. But her pain did not disappear, but rather seemed to worsen following the fusion surgery. When she came to our clinic, she was at the end of her tether. On detailed examination, we found that her pain was originating from the sacroiliac joint and not the spine as such.

We confirmed the diagnosis of SI joint disease through imaging and then proceeded to treat her with anti-inflammatory injections. The relief from pain was miraculous indeed! We followed up with a multidisciplinary treatment plan, which included physical therapy and a weight loss regimen. It is clear in Mrs. Murthy's case that the dual factors of delay in seeking treatment plus improper/wrong advice led to her suffering from chronic pain for so many years.

The longstanding pain had seriously impacted her quality of life as well.

Facet Joint Disease

When we refer to arthritis, invariably the weight-bearing joints in the lower limbs such as the knee and the hip joints come to mind, due to the high level of awareness about these structures among the common people.

This is because a tremendous amount of research has gone into the subject over the last two decades with immense advances in its management. Facet joint arthritis can be equally disabling, but it is not as well known or understood.

Here, there is arthritis occurring in the joints of the backbone. Facet joint disease can affect the cervical, thoracic, and lumbar vertebrae, but for now, we will focus on the lumbar segment as this is more commonly affected.

Anatomy: The vertebral bones are the building blocks of the spine and the facet joints connect adjacent vertebrae. Each vertebra has a superior articulating process and an inferior articulating process, which contribute to the joint above and below, respectively. These are true synovial joints, which are lined by articular cartilage. They have synovial fluid to promote lubrication of the joint surface and are covered by a capsule.

Function: The facet joints facilitate forward flexion and twisting movements of the spine by allowing the articular surfaces to glide over each other. They also contribute to the stability of the spine by preventing excessive movement in some other planes, such as extension.

Innervation: Facet joints are known to have dual innervation. In the lumbar spine region, the facet joint is innervated by the medial branch that arises from the dorsal ramus at the same level and the medial branch from the nerve one level above.

Causes:

(1) Traumatic degeneration of the facet joints. The facet joint may be affected following a primary injury such as a road traffic accident or a fall from a height.

(2) Age-related or mechanical degeneration of the joints. Degenerative changes in joints of the spine are inevitable as one ages.

Attention needs to be given to these changes when they lead to pain or disability.

(3) Occupational hazards. People in certain occupations are more likely to develop facet joint disease; for example, laborers who have been carrying heavy weights on their head and shoulders for many years.

Symptoms:

1. Low back pain which is of a deep, dull aching character. The pain is generally limited to the back and the buttock region, and the characteristic radiating pattern of pain seen in sciatica is not usually found here. However, in advanced cases of facet joint involvement, bone spurs can impinge on the respective nerve root giving rise to radiating pain. This presents a confusing picture and the physician should be careful while making the diagnosis to differentiate it from sciatica.

2. Aggravated by standing for long periods. The patient may find it difficult to get up after sitting for a prolonged time as well. Early morning stiffness is described in some cases. Twisting movement of the backbone can also bring on the pain.

3. Relieved by bending forward. People with facet joint disease usually prefer a hunched position as bending forward relieves the pain.

4. Facet joint involvement in the cervical and thoracic segments can produce pain and stiffness in the neck, shoulders, and upper and mid-back regions.

Signs:

1. Tenderness on extension and lateral bending of the spine.

The examining doctor can elicit pain when the patient bends backward or bends sideways.

2. Paramedian tenderness and paraspinal muscle spasm as the muscles go into a protective spasm to reduce the pain. The muscles close to the spine or parallel to the spine will be painful to touch and may also feel hard and bunched up.
3. Shopping Cart Sign. The patient may adopt the posture of bending over a shopping cart to relieve the pain. This happens when the facet arthropathy is very advanced and leads to narrowing of the intervertebral foramen causing spinal stenosis.

Diagnosis:

(a) Imaging: X-ray oblique view and CT and MRI scans can not only point toward the diagnosis of facet joint disease but also help in excluding other red flag indications of the spine. Red flag indications refer to other possible diagnoses that can be made for the presenting symptoms.

(b) LA injection: The most reliable test is an injection of LA into the joint or into the nerves supplying the joint. If the pain is not relieved, it is unlikely that the pain is coming from the facet joints.

Treatment:

1. Conservative: Our common painkillers, also known as nonsteroidal anti-inflammatory drugs (NSAIDs), have been used to control the flare-up of pain. There are other supportive measures that may help such as rest, spine strengthening exercises, hydrotherapy, and traction. Some patients reported that they have experienced considerable pain relief following osteopathic and chiropractic manipulations. This is a nonsurgical modality of treatment for people suffering from back pain, and the manipulations are called "adjustments."

2. Interventional: When conservative measures don't provide relief, interventional pain management comes into play.

   A mixture of an LA and a steroid preparation is injected around the nerves supplying the joint (medial branch block) or directly into the joint itself. Because the facet joints have a peculiar nerve supply, injection of LA into one joint can have an effect on the facet joints at two or three other levels as well. This procedure is said to be diagnostic as well as therapeutic as mentioned earlier. Blocking of the nerves is preferred nowadays to injecting into the joint.

3. Regenerative Medicine: In regenerative medicine, damaged and diseased tissues and cells are replaced or repaired using stem cells or tissue engineering. Platelet-rich plasma (Prp) and stem cells have been used by some study centers to prevent the progression of arthritis, but the efficacy of these procedures is yet to be proven in large-scale studies.

4. RF ablation or Rhizotomy of the medial branches supplying the facet joint can be considered in those patients who have a relapse following successful treatment with injections into the joint. In rhizotomy, the sensations are removed from painful nerve fibers by severing them with a surgical instrument or burning them using chemicals or electric cautery. In RF ablation the electrical conduction of the nerve fibers is destroyed using the heat emanating from a medium frequency alternating current source.

5. Surgery: Facetectomy and foraminotomy are the two surgical procedures that can be performed to increase the dimension of the intervertebral foramen and achieve adequate decompression of the affected nerve root. Fusion of two or more vertebrae is carried out as a final attempt to prevent movement at the affected level, thereby eliminating pain in the joint.

Prevention:

(a) Elimination of the cause. For instance, a manual

laborer with early symptoms can avoid lifting heavy weights and do some lighter work to prevent the progression of the disease.

(b) Exercises to strengthen the spine and increase mobility. People should be encouraged to take up some regular physical activity such as yoga, Pilates, aerobics, or athletics, or whatever else suits them.

(c) Watch your weight. Obesity is known to exacerbate facet joint disease and overweight people should be encouraged to reduce their weight to prevent the development of this condition.

Differential Diagnoses:

1. Sacroiliac joint disease
2. Disc Prolapse/Migration
3. Ankylosing Spondylitis
4. Piriformis syndrome
5. Endometriosis
6. Myofascial Pain
7. Hip Pain

Piriformis Syndrome

Introduction: In this condition, the piriformis muscle either goes into a spasm, thereby causing pain in the buttock region, or the muscle irritates the sciatic nerve, leading to pain similar to that caused by true sciatica. This condition is also referred to as wallet neuritis or deep gluteal syndrome. It is six times more common in women than in men.

Anatomy: The piriformis muscle[2] (PM) extends from the lower end of the spine (pelvic surface of S2—S4 sacral vertebrae) and passes through a large foramen called the greater sciatic notch to get

---

[2]https://www.physio-pedia.com/Piriformis

attached to the upper surface of the thigh bone (greater trochanter of the femur) on either side. The PM is functionally involved with external rotation, abduction, and partial extension of the hip. The sciatic nerve is the largest nerve in the human body and it generally exits the pelvis below the belly of the muscle; however, many congenital variations may exist.

For instance, it may either pass through the PM or pass above it. Due to these variations, there is a chance of irritation to the sciatic nerve.

Causes:
1. Muscle spasm in the PM can cause irritation of the sciatic nerve. Muscle spasms of the PM are most often caused by direct trauma, post-surgical injury, and lumbar and sacroiliac joint pathologies or overuse.
2. Hematomas (blood collection outside a blood vessel) can form in the PM after a fall on the buttock and this can irritate the sciatic nerve.
3. Swelling and tightness can occur in the PM as a response to injury or spasm.
4. Scar tissue that is formed after healing of an injury to the PM is usually not very flexible and can irritate the sciatic nerve.
5. Certain activities can cause spasms in the PM: prolonged sitting on a hard surface with a wallet in the back pocket, exercise on a hard and irregular surface, exercise after a long period of lay off.

Symptoms:

1. Sciatica with radiating pain starting from the buttocks going along the back of the leg to the outer border of the foot.
2. Buttock pain, which is of a dull achy character.
3. Associated tingling and numbness. Weakness in lower limbs or reduced sensation is quite rare.

4. Sitting is particularly painful and difficult, and patients tend to raise the affected buttock a little higher while sitting.
5. The pain is aggravated on adduction and internal rotation and it usually lessens when the patient is lying down, bending the knee, or walking.

Signs:

There are a number of signs that the physician can elicit to confirm the diagnosis of piriformis syndrome:

1. FADIR test: This stands for Flexion, Adduction, and Internal Rotation. If the patient develops sciatic pain on performing these three movements, the FADIR test is said to be positive and points to the irritation of the sciatic nerve by the PM.
2. PACE test: Here the patient is made to perform abduction and external rotation of the hip against resistance in a sitting position. The test is said to be positive if the patient experiences pain and weakness.
3. FREIBERG sign: Forced passive internal rotation of the hip joint when lying down can result in pain and weakness, and this points to passive stretching of the PM causing pressure on the sciatic nerve.
4. Gluteal tenderness: Deep palpation with the fingers in the gluteal region can elicit tenderness.
5. Per rectal examination: Digital rectal examination can cause pain similar to the patient's symptoms.

Differential Diagnosis:

The diagnosis of piriformis syndrome is based mainly on the clinical history and the presenting signs and symptoms.

There are many conditions that can mimic the presentation of piriformis syndrome.

- Sciatic neuropathy
- Lumbar disc herniation
- Sacroiliac joint inflammation or dysfunction
- Post-laminectomy syndrome
- Posterior facet syndrome at the lower lumbar and sacral vertebral levels
- Sacroiliac joint pain
- Trochanteric bursitis
- Pudendal nerve entrapment
- Unrecognized pelvic fractures

Investigations:

X-ray imaging is not very helpful. In some patients, nerve conduction studies and MRI can help point to the diagnosis on correlation with clinical findings, but these are not always helpful.

An injection of local anesthetic under USG or fluoroscopy is considered the most definitive means of diagnosis.

Treatment:

Initially, the patient is advised rest, and NSAIDs and muscle relaxants are used. Physical therapy has a very important role as many cases can resolve with focused exercises. The methods that are used are Ultrasound massage and Deep Tissue Release techniques with a structured program for piriformis and hamstring stretches.

Patients who do not respond to these methods can opt for USG- or Fluoroscopy-guided injections of LA+steroid.

Prolotherapy with fenestration on subsequent sittings also helps patients with piriformis syndrome. BOTOX preparations can also be used in certain patients who do not show any improvement in their symptoms with the other treatments. Botox acts by causing functional denervation of the muscle and relieving the spasm.

Surgical options include the release of the tendon at the attachment on the greater trochanter, dissection through the piriformis muscle, or neurolysis of the sciatic nerve.

Prevention:

Patients with piriformis syndrome can follow a few tips to prevent their symptoms from worsening:

1. Avoid sitting for prolonged periods, especially at work or while driving. Take frequent breaks to walk around and stretch your legs.
2. Be careful to continue with the home stretching exercises regularly.
3. Avoid activities that are likely to hurt the gluteal muscles such as sitting on a bulky wallet.

We have seen a few of the conditions that can cause chronic back pain. Let me share the story of Mr. Gopidas, who came to us with a history of back pain. What was behind his pain?

CASE STUDY 7

Mr. Gopidas was a hardworking postman who took his work very seriously. He never took a day off and one could see him riding his bicycle and diligently delivering the post in his area every day. He had been having pain for the last seven to eight years in his lower back.

And because his profession involved being on the move constantly, he did not neglect the pain. He consulted various doctors and was diagnosed as having conditions ranging from muscle spasms to disc problems.

He underwent many rounds of physiotherapy and he also made a visit to a neighboring state on the advice of some of his friends, to a place that specialized in massage therapy. All to no avail; he did not find any relief from his pain.

When Gopidas came to our clinic we took a detailed history, which included the history of his occupation. After thoroughly examining him, we were able to figure out that it was the cycle seat that was behind his pain! We found that it was an old seat, a bit lumpy in places, and not very comfortable.

Gopidas also carried his wallet with him in his back pocket constantly. Here are two contributing factors for the pain that had been overlooked so far! See how important it is to take a thorough history and make a careful examination of the patient! In this case, it helped us make the diagnosis of Piriformis Syndrome.

Gopidas was treated with image-guided BOTOX injections and advised some stretching exercises. He was soon relieved of 80 percent of his pain and began to feel much better. We advised him to change his cycle seat, and also follow some other steps in his occupation to ensure that there was no recurrence of the pain.

Intervertebral Disc Diseases

Anatomy:

The intervertebral discs are cushion-like structures situated between adjacent vertebral bones. They help in connecting the vertebral bones to each other. The three main components of the disc are nucleus pulposus, annulus fibrosus, and cartilaginous endplates. The cartilaginous endplates are the sole source of blood supply to the intervertebral disc.

Innervation is by a nerve called the sinovertebral nerve. The disc is made up of water and collagen and elastin fibers. The intervertebral disc acts as a shock absorber for the body and prevents the vertebral bones from grinding against each other. The structures around the vertebral bodies that can be affected by disc diseases are ligamentum flavum, the facet joints, and the shape of the neural foramina.

Types of disc problems:

1. Disc strain: Sometimes carrying heavy loads for extended periods of time may cause irritation or inflammation of the disc leading to pain. This will usually resolve with rest and if required mild analgesics may be used.
2. Disc herniation: You may come across many terms like slipped disc, disc bulge, and disc herniation, protrusion, or extrusion. Technically, they are different levels of the same pathology.

    Here, basically, there is a weakened area in the outer shell of the disc through which the soft spongy jelly-like material oozes out. When this material comes in contact with nearby spinal nerves, it can cause radiating pain as well as altered sensation. Disc herniation is most commonly seen in the lumbar vertebrae, and therefore the pain is mostly referred to the legs.
3. Disc degeneration: The water content of the intervertebral discs decreases with age. As we grow older, the disc becomes thinner and this can lead to friction between adjacent vertebral bones. This friction can lead to bony growths called bone spurs. This condition is seen mainly in older people and the pain may be aggravated by prolonged sitting or activity.

Treatment:

Most disc problems resolve with adequate rest. Mild pain relievers like Paracetamol or NSAIDs may be used.

Heating pads can be used to help reduce inflammation. Gentle massage is also helpful.

Sciatica

Sciatica is the condition where the pain is caused by irritation, inflammation, or compression of the sciatic nerve. The pain arises from the spine and typically radiates down through the buttocks and back of the leg.

Causes:

1. Herniated disc: This is the commonest cause of sciatica pain. The herniated disc in the lower back region can compress the sciatic nerve, leading to shooting pain.
2. Spinal stenosis: Certain conditions like osteoarthritis, thickened ligaments, tumors, or spinal injuries can cause narrowing of the foramina in the vertebrae, thereby leading to compression of the nerves that are traveling through them. Spinal stenosis occurs most commonly in the cervical (neck) and lumbar (lower back) regions. When the lumbar vertebrae are affected, the sciatic nerve is compressed.
3. Spondylolisthesis: Here, one vertebra slips out of alignment and this leads to narrowing of the foramen and pinching of the nerve.
4. Trauma, tumors, and Piriformis syndrome are some of the other conditions that can cause sciatic nerve compression.

Symptoms:

1. Moderate to severe pain in the lower back and buttocks that radiates down the backside of the leg. It is usually unilateral, but in rare cases, can be bilateral as well.
2. Weakness of the muscles in the lower back, legs, or feet on the affected side.
3. The pain may worsen on commencing movement or activity and subside on rest.
4. There may be altered sensations felt in the legs and feet

such as tingling, 'pins and needles,' or numbness.

5. In a rare condition called Cauda Equina syndrome, the affected person may lose bowel and bladder control as well.

Diagnosis:

(a) Physical examination: The physician will test muscle strength and muscle reflexes. The patient might also be asked to perform stretching and moving exercises to find out what activities increase the pain.

(b) Imaging: X-ray imaging can help in detecting the narrowing of the spinal canal or the presence of bony spurs. MRI and CT scans can help in the detection of sciatic nerve damage. CT myelogram, where a special dye is injected into the spinal cord, can be performed to get clear images of the spinal cord and the nerves.

(c) Nerve conduction studies: Also known as electromyography, this helps in studying how fast the electrical impulses travel through the affected nerve and also how the muscles innervated by the sciatic nerve respond to the stimuli.

Treatment:

1. Hot/cold compress: In the early stages of sciatic pain, the use of ice packs and heating pads is known to help. It is recommended to start with the cold pack and apply it to the painful areas for about 10 to 20 minutes at a time. After a couple of days, when the swelling has come down, you can start using heating pads. Always remember to wrap the pads in a towel before using them. Alternating between ice and heat therapy is known to be helpful in managing sciatica.

2. Stretching exercises: Gentle stretching exercises performed under the guidance of a physical therapist can be beneficial in relieving sciatica pain.

3. Pain relief medications: NSAIDs can help in reducing pain, inflammation, and swelling. All medications should be taken only on advice from your treating physician. In case of severe pain, your physician might prescribe muscle relaxants or narcotic pain killers.

4. Regular exercise: Staying active can be helpful in relieving pain. Consult your physician or physical therapist before undertaking any activity. You can start with some low-impact activities such as stationary cycling or swimming.

5. Epidural injections: When the pain does not decrease with the above methods, epidural steroid injections may be given. The epidural space is the gap between the vertebral body and its covering called the dura mater. Anti-inflammatory medication such as steroids when injected in this space help in reducing inflammation and pain.

6. Surgery: Surgery is advised only in cases of severe pain or weakness. Procedures such as discectomy or microdiscectomy are performed. This basically involves removing the portion of the intervertebral disc that is impinging on the sciatic nerve.

Prevention:

There are a number of things one can do to prevent the development or exacerbation of sciatica.

1. Posture: Maintaining proper posture while sitting, lifting heavy weights, standing, and sleeping will ensure that there is no extra stress applied to the spine. Avoid sitting or standing for prolonged periods of time.
   Always change your position at the first hint of discomfort.

2. Weight: Maintaining a healthy body weight is very important in reducing stress to the spine. Those who are overweight

will find a definite improvement in their symptoms when they begin to lose weight. The spine experiences the least stress at the ideal body weight.

3. Smoking: Nicotine is said to reduce the blood supply and thus weaken the spine and the vertebral discs. Avoiding smoking can reduce stress on the spine.

4. Exercise: Regular exercises can keep the muscles of our lower back and abdomen supple and strong. Healthy muscles provide good support to the spine.

To summarize, the backbone or the spine plays a crucial role in support and maintenance of the erect posture, while at the same time lending extensive flexibility to perform movements such as bending down or twisting sideways.

A healthy backbone is essential for a person to perform his normal daily activities and chronic pain can seriously impact the quality of life. Just as the owner of a building or house takes care in maintaining his property, and seeks to resolve a problem before it can damage or weaken the structure, the spine too must be taken care of. Symptoms of pain or limitation in movement should be investigated immediately.

The key is to seek early help at the right source. Knowledge of the structures that can generate pain in the backbone and the diseases that can affect it will help you easily convey your symptoms to your physician, in turn helping them to arrive easily at the correct diagnosis. The right treatment at the right time is the key to a pain-free life.

Precepts and Precautions

1. Maintain proper posture while sitting and standing.
2. Use a chair that provides adequate support to the back: Ergonomic chair.
3. Maintain ideal body weight.
4. Perform back-strengthening and stretching exercises regularly.

5. Avoid lifting heavy objects. If you have to lift something heavy, follow the correct method: bend the knees and keep the back straight.
6. Stop smoking: smoking decreases blood flow to the spine, and smokers are more prone to back pain.
7. Choose a comfortable sleeping posture. Use a pillow under your thighs/knees if you are sleeping on your back.
8. Invest in a firm mattress that provides good support to your spine.
9. Take frequent breaks if your job involves sitting in one position for a long time.
10. Avoid wearing high-heeled footwear.

5

PAINFUL CONDITIONS IN THE NECK

It is definitely a pain in the neck!

Everyone has at some time or the other experienced pain in the neck region. In fact, the commonly used idiom "a pain in the neck," which refers to something or someone who is being a constant source of irritation or disturbance is an indication of how much literal pain in the neck regions can affect us. The discomfort, distress, and hardship that a person suffering from neck pain undergoes is quite a lot.

Pain anywhere in the body, particularly if it is longstanding, can have a huge impact on a person's life. So much more so, if the pain is in the head and neck regions. Chronic neck pain can have a debilitating effect on a person's life. It can reduce your ability to enjoy life, socialize, do productive work, and sleep well. Neck pain has indeed been recognized as one of the leading causes of disability in people.

Not only does it cause physical disability and limitations, but painful conditions in the neck can also have a huge impact on your mental well-being. People with chronic neck pain have been known to suffer from psychological conditions such as anxiety and depression. Especially when a proper diagnosis is not made and patients are told that they are either imagining their pain or exaggerating it, it can be very depressing and disheartening for them.

The Upper Story

We saw how the backbone or spine can be compared to a multistorey building while speaking of chronic back pain. If the lower part of the spine can be compared to the basement, then the upper vertebral bones represent the upper floors of the same building! And just as disruption or damage to the basement can destabilize a building, anything that weakens the upper stories can lead to instability as well.

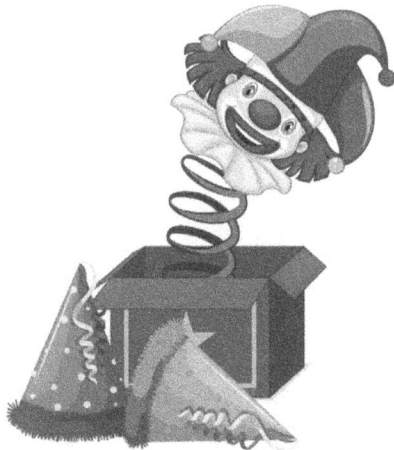

The upper part of the spine, or the cervical spine, can be compared to a tightly coiled spring that we see in machines. The different rounds of coils in the spring may be compared to the different intervertebral discs. The role of such a spring is mainly to act as a shock absorber. It also compresses and relaxes as required when pressure is applied.

When the coil loses its elasticity, then its action is lost as well. The cervical vertebrae not only act as shock absorbers but also help in the movements of the neck. The other parts present around the coiled spring help to stabilize it and hold it in place for its optimum action. In the same way, to stabilize the movements at the neck, there are various ligaments present that support the backbone. Otherwise, your neck might be popping about like the proverbial Jack-in-the-Box. We know that there is a lot of movement that happens in the neck regions:

(a) Flexion: Bending forwards with chin to the chest
(b) Extension: Bending backward, looking up at the sky
(c) Rotation: Turning head to the right or the left
(d) Side-bending: Tipping the head sideways to touch the shoulder with the ear

Just as the integrity of the coil is essential to the smooth running of the machine, a healthy spine allows pain-free movements in the body. The cervical spine carries out a lot of flexion–extension movements over the years. It is inevitable that there is some wear-and-tear happening all the time. When the structures related to the backbone are weakened, it may lose its curvature or its proper alignment. This can lead to changes in the way it works, which in turn can cause degenerative changes. The degenerative changes that occur over time can lead to disc herniation, and in later stages, cause instability as well.

Anatomy:

The cervical spine region consists of the upper 7 vertebral bodies. They are named C1 to C7. C1 vertebra connects to the skull bone and is called Atlas. C2 vertebra is called as Axis. They not only play a role in neck movements but also help protect the upper part of the spinal cord and the nerves that are going from the spinal cord to the upper limbs.

They also help in the attachment of muscles that move the shoulders. The cervical spine supports the weight of the head as well. Another important feature that is present only in the vertebral bones C1—C6 is a small opening that allows the vertebral arteries to carry blood to the brain.

Just reading the list of activities that depend on the cervical spine gives us an idea of how important it is. Unfortunately, this knowledge about the cervical spine and the various structures in and around it that can commonly be affected is very limited.

Owing to this reason, many people with chronic neck pain remain undiagnosed for many years and continue to suffer. What are the structures in the neck that may be affected leading to chronic neck pain?

1. Muscles: Muscles in the neck help to support the head and also aid in the movements of the head. Some of the main muscles are the sternocleidomastoid, trapezius, and suboccipital muscles. Sometimes, due to poor posture, trauma, or accident, the neck muscles may be injured.

2. Ligaments: The three main ligaments present in the cervical region are the anterior longitudinal ligament (ALL), the posterior longitudinal ligament (PLL), and the ligamentum flava. The ligaments in the spine help in connecting adjacent vertebrae. They too play a role in the movements of the head and neck. They can be affected by sharp trauma causing a tear or when sudden movement beyond the normal range occurs.

3. Vertebral bone: The vertebral bone per se may be affected in trauma and accidents causing fractures. Sometimes dislocation of a joint can occur, especially in the atlantoaxial joint.

4. Intervertebral disc: The intervertebral disc plays a major role in cushioning shock in the spine. The disc may undergo rupture, degeneration, herniation, etc.

5. Joints: The intervertebral joints can be affected.

As in the lower back, the facet joints are mainly affected in the cervical spine too. There may be fractures, degeneration, arthritic changes, etc., in the joint.

6. Nerves: There are eight paired cervical nerves that exit through the seven cervical vertebrae. These nerves provide innervation to the neck, shoulders, arms, and hands. These nerves can become irritated or compressed by the adjacent bony structures, ligaments, or intervertebral discs. This leads to motor and sensory dysfunction in the affected areas.

Let us now see the specific conditions that can bring on chronic neck pain.

1. Sprains and Strains

These mainly occur in the muscles and the ligaments that are present in the cervical region. Following trauma or a fall, or bad posture for a long time, the muscles in the spine may be stretched severely or they may even tear. This may lead to inflammation and swelling in the affected muscle, with limitation of movement and severe pain on movement. Muscle and soft tissue injuries often accompany whiplash trauma. Ligament injuries in the cervical spine are commonly caused by road traffic accidents or sports injuries.

The ligaments may stretch, twist, or even tear following trauma. When this happens, the muscles present close to these ligaments try to compensate and this leads to painful muscle spasms.

Prolonged poor posture can lead to increased strain on the ligaments and muscle fatigue. Symptoms: Severe pain, tenderness, bruising, swelling, stiffness and soreness, loss of movement, etc.

Investigations and Diagnosis:

Following trauma, X-ray imaging can help rule out fractures.
MRI within 72 hours of trauma helps in pointing to ligament injury.

In longstanding cases, instability of the spine can help in the diagnosis.

Treatment:

In acute cases, immobilization, use of hot packs, local application of pain gels, anti-inflammatory drugs, and bed rest may help to resolve symptoms. In longstanding cases, the use of cervical collars is advocated. Massage therapy and physical therapy can help reduce the pain and improve movement at the affected site. In some cases of ligament tears, surgery is indicated.

2. Cervical Spondylosis

This condition affects the intervertebral joints in the cervical spine. In cervical spondylosis, due to aging and wear and tear, the intervertebral disc slowly hardens due to loss of water or dehydration. This eventually makes the disc rigid and leads to degenerative changes.

As the size of the disc decreases due to all these changes, there is extra bony growth to compensate. These growths are called bone spurs, and when they rub against each other during movement, pain occurs.

3. Cervical Spondylitis

This may be the condition most people are familiar with. Any neck pain is usually termed cervical spondylitis in general. What exactly happens in spondylitis? Here too, the intervertebral joints are affected.

Spondylitis usually occurs as a result of inflammatory changes. These changes can lead to arthritis of the joint. One common autoimmune inflammatory condition is rheumatoid arthritis. Sometimes as these inflammatory changes progress, the joints start losing their mobility and can become fused to each other. This condition is called Ankylosing spondylitis.

Symptoms:

Both conditions present with many common symptoms. The main symptoms are pain, limitation of movement, stiffness, muscle spasm, etc. Spondylosis usually presents in the older age groups. Patients with cervical spondylosis in advanced condition may present with tingling sensation and numbness in the arms and hands, difficulty in walking and coordination, or loss of bladder and bowel control.

Investigations and Diagnosis:

Cervical spondylosis can be diagnosed in many patients based on the history of their condition and a thorough physical examination by the doctor. Imaging modalities such as X-ray spine, MRI, or CT scan can help in identifying disc degeneration, narrowing of disc space, bone spurs, and other bone abnormalities. Let us now see two important disease conditions that can arise out of these different degenerative, traumatic, or inflammatory states.

4.   Cervical Spondylotic Myelopathy (CSM)

CSM commonly affects the elderly. The term is self-explanatory.
- Cervical: Affects the neck region
- Spondylosis: Wear and tear changes are present
- Myelopathy: These changes affect the spinal cord.

As the term specifies, age as well as wear and tear changes in the spinal column or the vertebral structures damage the spinal cord. The spinal cord can be compared to the main power cable. It carries all the nerves to the different parts of the body from the brain. Messages to and from the different parts of the body are conveyed through different nerves, which may exit or enter the spinal column at different levels.

Conditions that can precipitate CSM are disc herniation, development of bone spurs, inflammatory diseases like rheumatoid arthritis, etc. In CSM, there is compression of the spinal cord. It is very important that this condition be diagnosed correctly and early; once the complications of CSM set in, it is usually a downhill journey for the patient.

Symptoms:

CSM does not have a sudden onset, but rather develops over time. The rate at which symptoms become severe may vary from person to person. In some people, it may take a very long time to manifest serious side effects. In others, the condition may worsen in just a few years. The main symptoms of PAIN and STIFFNESS will be present Apart from that, the patients may present with the following complaints.

(i) Muscle weakness that progresses over time. The shoulder and hand muscles usually get affected. The patient will not be able to lift their hands or arms. You can very well imagine how this can impact their daily life. They will be unable to carry things or have a grip on things.

(ii) When the sensory nerves are involved, the person can experience a tingling sensation all down his arms. They may also develop numbness or loss of sensation.

(iii) There may be difficulty experienced in walking and balancing.

(iv) Patients may present with loss of bowel and bladder control.

Diagnosis:

The doctor can suspect CSM in a patient based on their medical history, especially the presence of pre-existing medical conditions, and a thorough physical examination. Upper limb weakness can be a sign of CSM. The doctor may also be able to document the absence of sensations in the hands or the presence of muscle wasting.

MRI:

Myelopathy can be present in other conditions as well, such as multiple sclerosis or tumors in the spinal cord. MRI will help to confirm the diagnosis of CSM by showing the narrowing of the spinal canal caused by osteophytes or a herniated intervertebral disc.

CT scan and CT myelography: CT scans can help accurately assess spinal canal compromise. CT Myelography involves the injection of a contrast agent and this sometimes helps in planning the surgery.

Treatment:

Mild cases of CSM can be managed with conservative care such as the use of a cervical collar, physiotherapy to increase the strength of neck muscles, and pain-relieving medication when necessary.

When non-surgical methods fail to relieve the symptoms or when the patient has frank myelopathy, surgical management is the only choice. Cervical laminectomy or discectomy may be chosen for the patient depending on the specific condition of the patient. Some patients are treated with fusion surgery as a last resort to prevent the deformity from progressing.

5. Cervical Radiculopathy.

Cervical radiculopathy is a condition where the nerves roots or the nerves exiting from the seven cervical vertebrae may be affected. The nerves can be pinched or they may be inflamed. A single nerve root or multiple nerve roots may be involved depending upon the severity and extent of impingement or inflammation.

It is usually caused by a herniated intervertebral disc. It usually occurs in older people following degenerative changes in the disc. It can, however, occur in young people following trauma or when they have a spinal tumor.

The condition is seen to be a little more common in men than in women. The symptoms of cervical radiculopathy may not present all at once. They may appear intermittently in the initial stages of the disease. When it is a traumatic cause, then the symptoms can appear suddenly.

Etiopathogenesis: Degenerative Cervical Disc Disease: We have seen that the intervertebral disc has mainly three parts: the outer annulus fibrosis, the inner nucleus pulposus, and the cartilaginous endplates.

The nucleus pulposus is composed of a gel-like substance that is mainly composed of water, and as the person ages, the water content in the disc starts to decrease. Sometimes when this dehydration occurs at a rapid pace, the outer annulus fibrosis may develop defects or cracks. The intervertebral discs do not have a separate blood vessel supplying them. Much of the nutrients and oxygen reaches the parts of the disc by diffusion. Due to this reason, tears in the disc do not heal rapidly, or they heal with a weak scar that is susceptible to being injured again.

Traumatic Cervical Disc Migration: The cervical disc can migrate from its normal position and cause compression of nerve roots following sudden trauma, as in road traffic accidents, falls, or sports injuries.

Cervical Foraminal Stenosis: Narrowing of the foramen (opening through which a nerve will exit from the spinal cord) can cause the nerve traversing through to be impinged on. This can be caused by bone spurs that develop following degenerative changes in arthritis. Bulging of the disc or thickening of the ligaments in the spine can also cause compression of the nerve.

Foraminal stenosis is known to be the commonest cause of cervical radiculopathy.

Symptoms:

Pain: The main symptom experienced in cervical radiculopathy is radiating pain. The patient will describe sharp shooting pain that spreads from the neck to the shoulders and back and also the arms. The pain may extend right up to the hand and fingers. The pain is usually one-sided.

Altered sensations: Along with the pain, the patient may also complain of a tingling sensation or numbness along the affected arm. The patient may also notice weakness of the same limb.

Disc pain: When only the disc is involved like a bulging disc or a herniated disc, the condition may resolve on its own. But when there are bone spurs or a migrated disc causing the radiculopathy, spontaneous resolution does not happen. In these cases, it is advisable to treat as soon as possible

It is important to know how individual radiculopathies present.

(i)   C5 radiculopathy: Pain associated with tingling and numbness, radiating down from neck to shoulder, and down the arm till the thumb. There might be minimal weakness in the shoulder and upper arm.

(ii)   C6 radiculopathy: Pain radiates down to the index finger. Biceps muscle weakness may be present.

(iii)   C7 radiculopathy: Pain and other symptoms radiate down into the middle finger. Triceps weakness may be present.

(iv)   C8 radiculopathy: Pain and tingling radiate into the little finger. Handgrip strength may be reduced.

Diagnosis:

A thorough history from the patient usually helps in guiding the diagnosis toward cervical radiculopathy. History of unilateral pain is again important. Physical examination by the clinician involves detailed sensory and motor nerve evaluation.

This helps in localizing the level or the particular nerve roots involved in the radiculopathy.[3]

Nerve root	Muscle involved	Sensory deficits/location of pain	Reflex
C5	Deltoid	Lateral arm	Biceps
C6	Biceps, Wrist extension	Radial forearm, radial two digits	Brachioradialis
C7	Triceps, Wrist flexion	Middle finger	Triceps
C8	Finger flexors	Ulnar two digits	
T1	Intrinsic muscles of the hand	Ulnar forearm.	

There are some tests called provocative tests. Basically, in these tests, narrowing of the foramen is brought about to check if symptoms of cervical radiculopathy occur. Again, myelopathy should be ruled out. As we saw in the previous segment, in myelopathy, the patient can have an altered gait. Fine movements like writing or buttoning a shirt may be affected.

Sometimes along with cervical radiculopathy, the patient can also have peripheral nerve compression involving a specific nerve like the median nerve or the ulnar nerve. There may be overlapping of symptoms in such cases. Shoulder joint pathology must also be ruled out. Other diseases that can cause radiating pain, such as cardiac conditions and post–median sternotomy (post-surgery), must be kept in mind.

[3]https://www.ncbi.nlm.nih.gov/pmc/articles/PMC4958381/

Investigations:

(i)   X-ray cervical spine: To assess the disc height

(ii)   MRI: For soft tissue impingement and changes of myelopathy

(iii)   CT scan: To confirm bony involvement

Treatment:

Conservative treatment is tried first for maybe two or three months. If the patient finds no improvement, then surgical treatment might be attempted.

(a) Rest: The use of a cervical collar to restrict movement is advocated by some. The patient is advised to take adequate rest and also avoid strenuous activities like heavy lifting. The use of better posture for sitting and driving is advised.

(b) Physical Therapy: The patient may be advised by a trained physiotherapist about specific exercises and a stretching routine suitable for them. This may help improve neck and back strength and flexibility and thereby reduce pain. Any exercise should be started cautiously and increased gradually. Postural and ergonomic training may be included in this as well. Ergonomics simply means 'fitting the job to the person.' So, in this context, it would mean alterations suggested for the patient's workplace. For example, adjusting monitor height and keyboard placement, the use of a comfortable chair, and the facility to stand and work part of the time.

(c) Ice and/or heat therapy: Ice packs can help reduce pain. Sometimes warmth also helps. It is important to remember that applications should be limited to 15 or 20 minutes, which may be repeated if needed with an adequate two- to three-hour break in between.

(d) Cervical traction: In this process, the head is gently pulled up and this, in turn, helps to increase the space between the cervical vertebrae. This treatment was very popular previously. Now many clinicians do not use this as studies have shown it not to be beneficial.

(e) Manual manipulation: Many people undergo manual manipulation by a trained chiropractor. However, there are no corroborative studies to show that manipulation is beneficial in treating cervical radiculopathy in the immediate short-term or intermediate-term period.

(f) Medications: Mainly NSAIDs are used to control pain and inflammation in cervical radiculopathy. Sometimes oral steroids may be used to manage an acute inflammatory episode. Narcotic pain killers should be used with caution as their use may lead to dependence. Some patients benefit from muscle relaxants as well.

(g) Cervical epidural steroid injection: Corticosteroid injections can be given into the epidural space through image guidance. They provide relief by their anti-inflammatory effect as well as by decreasing the nociceptive (pain) stimulus

Surgical Treatment: When nonsurgical methods of treatment are not successful in addressing the pain or other symptoms, then surgical management can be considered.

The operations commonly performed are as follows:

- Anterior cervical discectomy with compression. A small incision is made in the front of the neck and the damaged or herniated disc is removed.

  The vertebrae are then fused with some graft material to maintain the height. This provides stability to the neck and at the same time allows the spinal nerves enough space without impinging on them.

- Cervical disc arthroplasty. In this procedure, after removing the damaged disc, an artificial disc is introduced instead of performing fusion of the vertebrae.
- Posterior decompression. Here the approach is through an incision made in the back of the neck. The surgeon will thin down the lamina, that is, the bony arch that forms the back of the spinal cord.

  This allows the surgeon to have better access to the compressed nerve. Any bone spurs or tissues that are compressing the nerve roots can now be cleared. Fusion of vertebrae is not performed here, and this allows quicker recovery and a better range of movement.

6. Cervical Facet Joint Syndrome

Osteoarthritis occurring in the cervical facet joints leads to a painful condition called Cervical Facet Joint Syndrome. The etiopathology of the condition is similar to that which we saw in facet joint disease in the lower back.

Causes: The main causes leading to facet joint disease in the cervical vertebrae are blunt trauma or whiplash injury. The other causes can be prolonged bad posture and aging.

Clinical features: Patients commonly complain of neck pain, headache, and limitation in neck movements. Dull aching pain may be present in the posterior neck that sometimes radiates to the shoulders or the mid-back regions. The person may have pain on touching the facet joints, pain on palpating the paraspinal muscles, or pain on extension or rotation of the neck. There may not be any gross neurological abnormalities seen.

Diagnosis: The diagnosis is mainly one of exclusion. Conditions that must be ruled out include cervical disc injuries, cervical discogenic pain, cervical radiculopathy, and cervical spine sprain/strain injuries. Imaging studies will help rule out the presence of fractures or tumors.

Treatment: Conservative treatment includes soft tissue massage, physical therapy, and posture correction. Some patients experience pain relief with anti-inflammatory medicines or muscle relaxants. A few others benefit from chiropractic adjustments. However, it is important that they must only consult qualified chiropractors and physiotherapists to avoid aggravating their condition with wrong manipulations.

For those with persistent pain, their doctors might prescribe facet joint injections with steroids or a medial branch block with a local anesthetic.

These procedures are performed under image guidance. Surgical treatment is rarely advocated in cervical facet joint disease. The results are not as good as those seen with surgery for radicular pain. Concomitant lifestyle changes may be recommended like losing weight, eating healthy food, regular exercising, and maintaining good posture.

As you can perceive, the painful conditions affecting the spine in the neck regions can be myriad. And when pain is neglected or the cause is not properly diagnosed, a downhill cascade can be set in motion leading to increasing pain as well as a decrease in mobility and range of motion. This in turn has a serious impact on the quality of life of the affected person. Dr. Meena Rajesh too underwent a lot of suffering before her condition was diagnosed correctly and she could receive the right therapy.

CASE STUDY 8

Dr. Meena Rajesh was a 42-year-old surgeon who came to us with a complaint of longstanding neck pain. She did not have any history of trauma to the neck except for a mild whiplash injury she suffered around 10 years before in a road traffic accident. In addition to the constant pain, she had various problems of tinnitus and drop attacks. Tinnitus is when you have a ringing sound in your ear constantly. Drop attacks are when a person just falls down all of a sudden without any external physical cause like getting tripped or pushed. They last for around 15 seconds and the patient quickly recovers.

She was investigated for various causes of tinnitus like a middle ear infection or inner ear damage. No cause could be identified for her drop attacks as well. She did not have any cardiac conditions, hypertension, or seizure disorders.

However, her symptoms continued to worsen over the years. She started having anxiety and panic attacks, always fearing she would fall unconscious. This sense of impending doom was a constant presence.

She consulted many orthopedic specialists and neurosurgeons. All investigations such as X-ray spine and MRI were performed a number of times. She was prescribed anti-inflammatory medications, which did not help her. She was constantly being told that there was nothing wrong with her, and she is imagining her symptoms.

On the advice of a relative, she consulted a traditional bone setter, who did manipulations and massage on her neck. To her alarm, she found a drastic worsening of her condition following this visit. She came to our clinic at this point, around eight years after her symptoms began. We noted the history of her complaints diligently and did a thorough evaluation.

We performed a DIGITAL DYNAMIC MOTION X-RAY of the spine. Our diagnosis was Facet Joint Degeneration with Cervical Instability. These occurred as sequelae to the whiplash injury that she had suffered 10 years before. At ALLEVIATE, we treated the facet joint disease with Platelet Rich Plasma (PrP).

Different levels of facet joints were treated. And the surrounding structures in the neck were given Prolotherapy. PROLOTHERAPY is now considered the 'go-to' treatment for cervical instability. Dr. Meena underwent four successive sessions of PrP + Prolotherapy in

4 months. At the end of 4 months, she experienced 70 percent to 80 percent resolution of her symptoms. She started feeling remarkably well, and her anxiety and sense of impending doom almost disappeared. She did not experience any further drop attacks. She also testified to a considerable reduction in neck pain. This was a story with a happy ending, fortunately. But there are numerous patients who continue to live with chronic neck pain simply because they have not been given the correct diagnosis. What exactly is cervical instability and why does it have such debilitating effects?

Cervical Instability

Cervical instability is a condition where there is excessive movement in the top two cervical vertebrae. This can occur because of laxity in the ligaments that connect these vertebral bodies to the skull. Ligament laxity may be due to many reasons, such as trauma, connective tissue disorders, or genetic causes. The commonest cause of trauma leading to ligament laxity is a whiplash injury. Whiplash injuries commonly occur in road traffic accidents, especially if one is not wearing a seatbelt. In a whiplash injury, the head and neck experience sudden forced backward movement followed by a lightning-quick forward movement. The cervical spine experiences an extreme amount of stress. The person can develop some immediate symptoms like neck pain, tingling in the arms, and shoulder pain.

However, most people with whiplash injuries will recover within a few months. Whiplash symptoms take a longer time to resolve in women and in older people. A severe whiplash injury can lead to extensive stretching of the spinal ligaments, leading to their laxity.

Why is it important to diagnose cervical instability correctly and early? Cervical instability can present with many symptoms:
- Headache
- Blurred vision
- Neck and shoulder pain
- Migraine

- Light sensitivity
- Tinnitus
- Dizziness
- Breathing difficulty
- Nausea
- Drop attacks
- Palpitations
- Brain fog
- Memory loss

Cervical instability can cause tension on the spinal cord, which in turn can pull on the brain and the brain stem. The nausea center is present in the brain stem and this is the reason why a person with cervical instability may feel nauseous all the time. In the same way, when the centers that control heart rate and blood pressure are affected, people with cervical instability can present with changes in the heart rhythm like tachycardia or hypotension.

There may be obstruction to the free-flowing of the cerebrospinal fluid, that is, the fluid flowing through the brain and the spinal cord. This free flow is essential to keep the brain and neurons healthy. In cervical instability, the patient will feel constant pressure in the head. Their vision may be affected. They will have trouble concentrating or remembering. This is called brain fog.

These are a few of the symptoms experienced by a person with cervical instability. Cervical instability can seriously impact the quality of life of the affected individual. Seeing the myriad ways in which it can affect a person definitely tells why it is important to recognize and treat this condition at the earliest.

Diagnosis: Diagnosis of the condition is based on history. Dynamic flexion and extension radiographs also help in the diagnosis to a large extent. MRI is said to have a limited role in the diagnosis of cervical instability that follows whiplash injury.

Treatment: The optimal treatment mode for each patient may vary depending on the cause of the instability, how long the patient has had the condition, and the presence of other comorbidities. The commonly employed methods are chiropractic treatment, physical therapy, strengthening exercises, and surgery.

Many people benefit from chiropractic manipulation for headache, spine misalignment, and poor posture that result from cervical instability. However, this must be attempted only by a qualified chiropractor. Physical therapy involving strengthening exercises, posture education, joint mobilization, soft tissue massage, and proprioception exercises are recommended. There are some specific strengthening exercises that are taught to the patient by a qualified physiotherapist.

Fusion surgery is sometimes undertaken in advanced cervical instability.

Prolotherapy

Prolotherapy is a relatively new treatment option for cervical instability. It is a regenerative technique whereby an injection is given to stimulate the body's natural healing process, which can help strengthen and repair injured joints and ligaments. It is especially helpful in longstanding cases of cervical instability. In this era of desk jobs requiring long hours peering at a computer screen, you must have heard of people complaining of various aches and pains.

And indeed, we have been studying a few of them here as well. However, Anirudh was suffering from neck pain for about 2 years now, and so far, none of the places he has gone for treatment have been able to help him. What could possibly be the matter? Let us find out.

CASE STUDY 9

Anirudh was a 32-year-old IT person who came to us with a history of neck pain that came on and off for the last two years. He did not have any history of injuries, trauma, falls, or being in a road traffic accident. He had been to see many doctors and all investigations had been done. Imaging like X-ray, CT scans, and MRI did not reveal any pathology in the spine or the joints.

He had been treated with anti-inflammatory medications, muscle relaxants, local application of cold and warmth, local pain applications like pain gels, and the list went on. He would sometimes get temporary relief with some of these treatments but the pain would always recur. Eventually, he was told that he just had a stiff back. One doctor told him his neck alignment was wrong, which alarmed him terribly. As the pain became chronic, he started getting depressed and demotivated.

When we saw him in our clinic, we were able to assess him and identify that he had multiple trigger points in the trapezius muscle. This is a large muscle that is present just below the skin and stretches from the base of the skull to the middle of the back. It also stretches sideways to both the shoulder blades. This gives it the appearance of a kite. He was treated with Trigger point injections, following which he experienced huge relief from pain. He underwent supervised physiotherapy and was taught some home exercises as well. Lifestyle modification was introduced with weight loss management advice as well as proper nutrition and diet planning from our nutritionist.

Workplace ergonomics was taken into account as well. Being in the IT field, he was sitting in one position for prolonged periods. He was advised about comfortable work furniture as well as maintaining correct posture while working. Anirudh was overjoyed with the drastic reduction in pain. He described his diagnosis and treatment at ALLEVIATE as a life-changing experience.

Cervical Trigger Points

Cervical trigger points are certain areas in the muscles of the neck, shoulders, and upper back that can be highly sensitive. They are painful to touch and can radiate pain to surrounding areas as well. Trigger points may occur following any muscle injury or they may even occur due to continuous muscle stress. Etiopathogenesis: The actual mechanism behind the occurrence of trigger points and the pain patterns associated with a particular trigger point is poorly understood. It has been proposed that acute muscle trauma or repetitive micro muscle injuries may cause muscle knots to form that are highly sensitive or irritable. Sometimes these trigger points develop over many years. Micro-trauma may be caused by lack of exercise, prolonged poor posture, sleep disturbances, or vitamin deficiencies. Any activity that causes repetitive stress on a specific muscle or muscle group can lead to the formation of trigger points. They may be sports-related or work-related activities.

Clinical Presentation:

The pain usually starts at a focal point and then in a matter of an hour or two, it spreads through the surrounding area. The pain can be quite debilitating and the patient may have decreased range of movement in the affected area. In the head and neck regions, this can present with headaches and eye pain. Sometimes muscles in the shoulder or upper limb may be involved. Trigger point pain can be a chronic condition seriously affecting the quality of life of the patient.

Diagnosis:

Usually, the condition is diagnosed by the clinician by palpating the muscle knot. It is felt as a tense or hard nodule in the muscle that is painful to touch. There may be a twitch response seen on the muscle. Palpation of the muscle knot can trigger the radiation of pain to the reference areas.

Treatment:

1. Massage therapy. Massaging by trained people may sometimes help relieve trigger point pain.
2. Physical therapy. Physical therapy with heat application and gentle stretching is said to be helpful.
3. Dry needling. Although the exact mode of action is not clear, injecting an empty needle into the trigger point and moving it around can relieve trigger point pain. Needling probably increases blood flow to the area and helps reduce muscle contraction.
4. Medications. Muscle relaxants have been helpful in reducing pain in a few patients.
5. Trigger point injections. Injections with a local anesthetic or just saline are given into the trigger point muscle. Sometimes steroids may be used as well. This makes the trigger point inactive and alleviates pain rapidly. The effect of anesthetic injections can last from a few weeks to a month. Steroid injections have a prolonged effect lasting up to several months.
6. Ergonomics. The patient's work environment and lifestyle need to be evaluated. Factors that could have contributed to the development of trigger points are identified. For those working at a sitting position, table height, chair height, and chair back support are some of the aspects that can be rectified.

The most important factor in the diagnosis of the cervical trigger point is the recognition of this condition. Most orthopedic surgeons neglect this condition as there is no surgical management for the same. Physicians and general practitioners too often overlook this diagnosis for the simple reason that they are not aware of its prevalence.

At ALLEVIATE, we are careful to get a comprehensive history from every patient. Once diagnosed, we treat cervical trigger points with ultrasonography. Image-guided dry needling or trigger point injections are given as required. We also take a multidisciplinary approach and take the person's lifestyle into account. Physical therapy is advocated. Lifestyle modifications like weight loss and proper diet are recommended. Ergonomics is also looked into for each patient. What work do they do? How is the work environment? What modifications can be helpful? These are some of the elements that we work on.

Cervical conditions are also poorly understood by doctors just as the other spine conditions are. Many conditions that are commonly seen go unrecognized, simply because the physicians assume that these conditions are not very common.

Only diseases of the disc are recognized and diagnosed early because it is a term that is commonly used. When a person presents with neck pain, we have to remember that it may be a disc problem, a facet problem, a trigger point, a muscle sprain, or a radiculopathy. We also should know what caused the condition, the aggravating factors, and the stage of the disease process. Being aware of these various conditions that can affect the neck region, can help in an accurate diagnosis. Do not allow it to remain a 'pain in the neck.'

Precepts and Precautions

1. Practice good posture while standing and sitting.
2. While traveling long distances or working for long hours at the desk, get up, move around, and stretch your neck and shoulders.
3. Ergonomics is vital—keep the monitor at your eye level. Knees should be positioned slightly lower than hips.
4. Avoid tucking the mobile between neck and shoulder while on a call. Use a headset instead, if your hands are not free.
5. Avoid carrying heavy bags with single shoulder straps.
6. Ensure that you sleep in a comfortable position. Use a small pillow for the neck. Sleep on your back with a pillow under the thighs. This flattens the spinal muscles and relax them.

7. Learn exercises to strengthen your neck and shoulder muscles.
8. Maintain ideal body weight.
9. Quit smoking—smoking is said to damage the structures in the spine and delay healing.
10. Do not neglect a pain in the neck region. It can lead to a decrease in mobility and range of motion.
11. Chronic neck pain can affect your quality of life.

6

FOOT AND ANKLE CONDITIONS

Wheels do matter

One of the very important but the least thought about parts of our body is our feet. No one spares them a thought unless they start sending distress signals. That is akin to the feet rebelling at the callous attitude with which they have been treated so far.

The feet help in locomotion; basically, they get you from one place to another. And being the lowermost part of the leg, they experience the maximum stress. It is said that in their lifetime, the average person walks anywhere up to 100,000 miles. That is a lot of walking! You can see how vital it is to ensure that your feet are healthy. Talking of moving, I would like to compare our feet to the wheels of a car or any vehicle. We all will agree that the wheels of a vehicle are a very important feature. They bear the entire load of the vehicle. In fact, they are the single feature without which a vehicle loses its very purpose for existence, namely, to transport people or goods from one place to another.

This is precisely why the owner of a car will always ensure that while servicing his vehicle, the wheels are checked out regularly too.

During its lifetime of service, a set of tires will have to bear different weights, travel varying distances, and traverse different kinds of terrain. The terrain might be a smooth road or a rough, rocky gravel path; it might be level ground or an incline uphill. This will give an idea of the amount of stress and strain experienced by the tires. A responsible owner will take care to check that the tire air pressure, wheel alignment, and tire treads are as they should be for optimal performance. Any deviation in these will be taken care of and rectified immediately.

In the same way, our feet have to serve us for a lifetime too. They have the role of bearing the weight of a person and carrying them around for their whole lifespan.

In our country, the awareness of foot and ankle health is very low. Most times people just ignore or put up with painful conditions of the feet and ankles. The general thinking is, "It is just the feet. Why bother?"

As long as the person is somehow able to manage and carry on with their daily activities, they will not pay much attention to pain in these areas. Only when the pain gets unbearable, or they are unable to walk or move, will they even agree to see a doctor. Unfortunately, most often, degenerative changes would have set in by this time or the damage would have become permanent, making the treatment all the more difficult. Moreover, people do not have an awareness of the different services and therapies that are available for treating foot and ankle conditions.

In developed countries, foot problems are looked into immediately because of good awareness about the services available. Here the main challenge is there are not many foot and ankle surgeons. Well-trained podiatrists too are not many, and this is why people, in general, are also not aware of podiatric services.

Coming back to our analogy, we know that there are different kinds of vehicles, for example, four-wheelers and two-wheelers, and the sizes of these vehicles differ too. For instance, a truck is a big vehicle, whereas a car is smaller. And it goes without saying that the tires needed for these vehicles differ too.

In the same way, the structure of the feet can differ in different people. The shape of the foot may vary or the structure of the foot arches may vary. Thus, it stands to reason that people need to wear footwear that is appropriate for their feet and structure.

Again, we can notice that the tires fitted to a vehicle also depend very much on the terrain that the vehicle is going to cross. For instance, there are snow tires if you live in a place that has snowfall, all-season tires for driving on the highway, and track and competition tires to be fitted in race cars. And it should be the same with footwear! Unfortunately, in our country, most people do not give so much thought to what they wear on their feet. Ill-fitting footwear and shoes can lead to many problems in the feet and ankle. It would be just like a person with a waist size of 34 inches squeezing into clothing sized 32 or 30 inches. You can imagine how uncomfortable that would be. In the same way, going about the whole day wearing unsuitable footwear can bring about a lot of discomfort to the feet and eventually lead to the development of chronic painful conditions.

Footwear must be chosen keeping many factors in mind: arch shape, gait pattern, the weight of the individual, hours of walking or standing they will be doing, to name a few. It is important to remember that bad or ill-fitting footwear in someone already predisposed to foot and ankle problems can accelerate the disease process, leading to degenerative changes and further damage.

Anatomy

The foot is a flexible part of our body that is attached to the leg at the ankle joint. The feet are involved in different actions such as walking, running, and jumping. The various structures present in the feet are bones, joints, muscles, and soft tissues like connective tissue, tendons, and ligaments.

It may surprise you to know that there are 26 bones and 33 joints in your feet. And the ankle joint comprises 3 main bones. The ligaments in the feet connect the different bones to each other, and the tendons connect muscles to the bones.

And all these elements need to function smoothly for a pain-free existence.

The foot can be divided into three parts: forefoot, midfoot, and hindfoot.

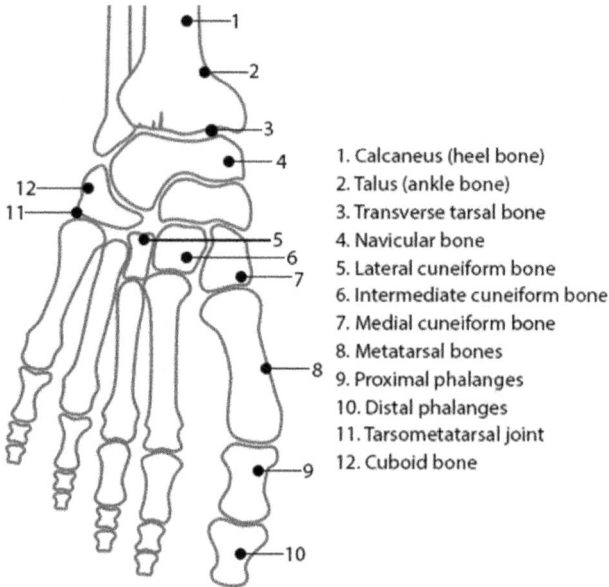

1. Calcaneus (heel bone)
2. Talus (ankle bone)
3. Transverse tarsal bone
4. Navicular bone
5. Lateral cuneiform bone
6. Intermediate cuneiform bone
7. Medial cuneiform bone
8. Metatarsal bones
9. Proximal phalanges
10. Distal phalanges
11. Tarsometatarsal joint
12. Cuboid bone

The forefoot comprises the five long metatarsal bones and five shorter bones called phalanges that form the toes. The five bones of the midfoot form the two arches. The hindfoot has two bones, talus and calcaneum. The talus connects with the tibia and fibula to form the ankle joint. The calcaneum is the largest bone in the foot and it forms the heel.

The various muscles, tendons, and ligaments work in tandem to help move the foot. The Achilles tendon is a well-known and important tendon that allows the calf muscles to move the ankle. All these together provide shape, flexibility, and strength to the foot.

Let us find out about the structures in the foot that can cause pain.

Bone: The bones in the feet may give rise to chronic pain in conditions like fractures, malunion or nonunion of bones, osteomyelitis, or tumors.

Muscles: Sprains and strains can occur in the muscles.

Soft tissues: The various ligaments and tendons can be affected by trauma or wear and tear.

Nerves: Some conditions like diabetes or nerve impingement can cause altered sensations in the foot called peripheral neuropathy.

What are the commonly seen painful conditions in the foot and ankle?

Ankle Instability

This condition can occur following long-standing sprains or repeated sprains in the ligaments of the ankle joint. It is most commonly referred to as the ankle giving way. This may happen when walking, or sometimes even while standing. When not treated properly, a simple sprain can quickly lead to progressive degeneration.

Symptoms: Pain, swelling, discoloration, loss of movement, sounds like popping or crackling, etc., may be present in the ankle joint. The person affected usually describes it as a wobbly or unstable feeling.

Diagnosis: Diagnosis of the condition is mainly based on the history of an old or repeated sprain on the affected side. X-ray and MRI can help detect bony and soft tissue involvement.

Treatment: Non-surgical Management. Physical therapy may be given to strengthen the ankle joint and improve its range of motion. Ankle braces are sometimes used to provide support to the ankle. Anti-inflammatory medications can help reduce pain and swelling in acute conditions. Surgical Management. Sometimes the surgeons will recommend repair and reconstruction of the damaged ligaments depending on the severity of the instability in the patient and the lifestyle of the patient.

Regenerative therapy: This is a new mode of therapy. In patients for whom degenerative changes have occurred in the joint, this is a boon. PROLOTHERAPY can help in regenerative restoration of joint function. It helps to repair the painful areas by stimulating healing. Prolotherapy may be combined with PrP and stem cell therapy also for better results.

Achilles Tendonitis

Achilles Tendon is the largest tendon in the body. It attaches the calf muscle to the heel bone. This tendon helps in movements of the foot such as walking, running, and jumping. The Achilles tendon can get damaged if there is prolonged use of the tendon or if there is repetitive intense strain applied to it. Moreover, this tendon can also weaken with age and become more susceptible to injury. Achilles tendonitis occurs more commonly in men. People with obesity or flat feet are also predisposed to develop Achilles tendonitis. The others in whom this condition can occur more frequently are sportsmen and athletes. Dancers, runners, and basketball and baseball players are some of those in whom the Achilles tendon gets repeatedly overstretched leading to damage and inflammation.

Symptoms: Achilles tendonitis can present as burning pain or stiffness above the heel bone. In the beginning stages, a mild ache may be felt in the back of the leg or above the heel. It usually appears after walking, running, or any sports activity. The calf muscles can feel tight and there may be a limited range-of-motion on flexing the foot. Severe pain can occur after prolonged walking, running, or climbing stairs.
In older people, there may be early morning stiffness and pain that may be relieved with mild activities. In chronic Achilles tendonitis, the patients will complain of soreness and pain on touching the area. In case of rupture of the tendon, the pain is sudden, intense, and severe.

Diagnosis: Doctors can differentiate this condition from an ankle sprain by thorough physical examination and checking the range of motion. In case of Achilles tendon rupture, the calf squeeze test will help in the diagnosis. Imaging modalities such as X-rays and MRIs can also help in diagnosing tendon damage.

Treatment: Conservative therapy. The RICE (rest, ice, compression, and elevation) method is recommended immediately following injury to the Achilles tendon. Rest without putting pressure on the affected side allows the tendon to heal faster.

The application of ice bags or cold compression can help in reducing inflammation and pain. A compression bandage can help reduce swelling, but it should not be applied too tightly. Elevation of the affected foot while lying down also helps in reducing the swelling.

Anti-inflammatory medication can also help in reducing inflammation and pain. Strengthening exercises and physical therapy are recommended once the acute inflammation and pain subside.

Surgical Management. When conservative treatment is not effective, surgical repair of the tendon may be necessary.

Prolotherapy. Prolotherapy has been found effective in patients with longstanding Achilles tendon pain. This is a non-surgical regenerative option of treatment. Patients receive injections, which are given under image guidance.

Plantar Fasciitis

The plantar fascia is a thick band of fibrous tissue that is present along the bottom of the foot. It extends from the heel bone to the toes. The plantar fascia functions as a support for the muscles and arches of the foot. It is shaped like a bowstring and absorbs the shock while walking. When this fascia is overstretched, tiny tears can occur in it.

Continuous stretching and tearing of the fascia can cause pain and inflammation. This condition is seen more commonly in women. Obesity and age above 40 can be predisposing factors for plantar fasciitis. It is also seen in runners and in those who wear footwear with inadequate support for the arches. Pregnancy is another condition where women can develop plantar fasciitis.

Symptoms: Typically, it is described as stabbing pain in the foot near the heel bone, which is at its worst in the first few steps taken after waking up. It can also occur when a person starts moving after prolonged periods of standing or sitting. Pain is increased after exercising (not during exercising). Tightness may be felt in the Achilles tendon.

Diagnosis: Physical examination by the doctor will reveal high arches in the feet. There may be pain on applying pressure to the bottom of the feet just in front of the heel bone. The pain will worsen when the patient points the foot upward (flexion) and decrease when the foot is pointed downward. X-ray imaging can help rule out other bony causes of heel pain such as fractures or arthritis.

Treatment: Conservative Management. Plantar fasciitis is generally considered a self-limiting condition. In most patients, the symptoms resolve by 6 to 18 months. Anti-inflammatory medications can help relieve pain and inflammation. Addressing some of the precipitating factors like badly fitting footwear and obesity can help in relieving pain and hastening the healing process.

Stretching and strengthening exercises can help in decreasing the tightness of the calf muscles and thereby relieve the pain. Night splints have been used at times to keep the foot in a neutral position while sleeping; this helps the plantar fascia to heal overnight in the elongated position and is said to reduce pain during the first steps in the morning.

Corticosteroid injections into the plantar fascia have been used. These must be administered only after ruling out other causes of heel pain by imaging studies. Steroid injections provide temporary relief, but eventually, the pain recurs in most cases.

Ice baths and ice massages have been advocated Precautions must be taken to avoid excessive exposure of the toes to cold.

Iontophoresis. Here low voltage electrical impulses are used to move local corticosteroids into the soft tissues. This treatment is usually reserved for athletes and sportspersons as well as people who are not able to carry out their professional activities.

Surgical Management. When pain is not relieved by conservative therapies, surgical release of the plantar fascia is performed.

Regenerative Therapy. Biological regenerative procedures such as Prolotherapy have been used to stimulate the body's natural ability to repair damaged tissue by promoting new growth. In our clinic, ALLEVIATE, we advocate three to four sessions of prolotherapy along with the administration of PrP. A multidisciplinary approach is taken in the treatment, and the patient is given support for physical therapy and weight management as well.

Ankle Sprain

Ankle sprains are probably the commonest injuries that occur in the foot. An ankle sprain occurs when the ligaments that support the ankle joint are overstretched and develop tears. The sprains can range from mild to severe depending upon the extent of the damage to the ligaments. Almost everyone has experienced an ankle sprain at some point in their lives.

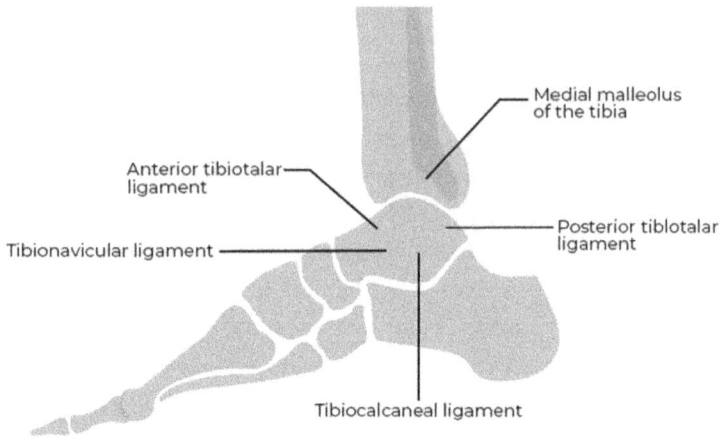

Medial malleolus of the tibia

Anterior tibiotalar ligament

Tibionavicular ligament

Posterior tiblotalar ligament

Tibiocalcaneal ligament

Most often they are minor injuries and the affected ligaments heal with rest and application of ice packs. At times there may be extensive tears in the ligaments that do not heal properly, or the ankle may sustain repeated strains. These conditions can lead to degenerative changes and ankle instability. Chronic ankle sprains are seen in sportspersons such as basketball players and footballers.

Ankle sprains can occur in the course of our normal life as well. For example, walking on an uneven surface or a badly paved sidewalk can cause the ankle to turn suddenly. Wearing high heels or footwear that does not provide adequate support to the feet can cause ankle sprains.

Symptoms: Pain and swelling are the commonest symptoms of a sprain. The ankle will be painful to touch and there may be increased warmth as well. The person may be unable to bear weight on the affected joint. Bruising may be seen around the sprained ankle. There may be stiffness in the joint. The range-of-movement will be decreased and there will be an increase in pain on attempted movements.

Diagnosis: The doctor will do a physical examination and check movements at the affected joint to get an idea of which ligaments might be injured. X-ray imaging will help rule out bone fractures at the ankle and MRI can help diagnose soft tissue damage to the joint and ligament tears. Ultrasonography allows the doctor to view the affected ligament while moving it. This helps in figuring out the extent of the damage.

Treatment: Ankle sprains are usually treated conservatively. Even some moderate sprains involving ligament tears will heal if the ankle is immobilized properly. The RICE protocol may be followed immediately following a sprain. Non-steroidal anti-inflammatory drugs may be used to reduce pain and inflammation. Crutches can be used to move around and avoid placing stress on the affected ankle. Immobilization of the ankle joint is advocated in cases of moderate or severe sprains to aid in the healing process. Splints or elastic crepe bandages may be used as per the clinician's advice.

Surgical therapy is undertaken only if there is severe damage to the ligaments and underlying ankle joint instability. Surgical management usually includes arthroscopy and reconstructive surgery. Arthroscopy is performed to check if there are any fragments of bone or cartilage in the affected joint. The orthopedic surgeon can repair the torn ligament with sutures, or other ligaments and tendons present in the ankle joint may be used for the reconstruction as well. Strengthening exercises help to strengthen the muscles around the affected ankle joint. It is important to do these exercises because even after the sprain has healed and the pain has disappeared, the ankle joint may not be very stable.

Preventing further sprains to the ankle is important. This can be achieved by supporting the affected ankle in crepe bandages, avoiding the use of high heels, walking carefully on uneven surfaces, and wearing sturdy and properly fitting footwear or shoes.

Regenerative Therapy: Conservative management of ankle sprains sometimes requires a long healing period. Some patients may have sprains that are causing nagging pain for more than six months duration. Some degenerative changes will most likely also have set in by this time. This will lead to ankle instability. Therapy with PrP is said to stimulate healing in the damaged tissues. It can help tighten lax ligaments in the affected ankle joint as well.

Hallux Valgus

They are commonly known as bunions. This is a bump or swelling that is seen on the outer surface of the big toe. This happens because the big toe deviates in, toward the second toe. This is a progressive condition. The first toe joint or the first metatarsophalangeal (MTP) joint is affected. This condition is seen more commonly in women and older people. The normal angle between the bones that form the first MTP is less than 15°, but in hallux valgus, the angle may be more than 20°. An angle of 45°–50° is considered to be a severe deformity. People who are born with structural deformities in the foot, like flat feet, are more likely to develop bunions. Also, there may be a family history of hallux valgus or the person may have rheumatoid arthritis. Wearing narrow footwear and standing for long periods of time can make the condition worse.

Symptoms: A small swollen bump is seen on the outer side of the big toe. The big toe will be turned toward the second toe, or it may even cross over the second toe. There will be pain in the first MTP joint. The patient may complain of pain in the ball of the first toe. The person may find it difficult to wear regular shoes.

Diagnosis: Most of the time, the condition is evident from external appearance. X-ray imaging of the foot will help the surgeon to know the extent of the deformity and identify the changes that have occurred in the joint. An angle greater than 20 degrees between the first metatarsal and the proximal phalanx of the first toe is diagnostic of the condition.

Treatment: Conservative Therapy: Mild cases of hallux valgus are usually treated with targeted exercises and physiotherapy. Patients may be prescribed special shoes or bunion splints to wear at night. In severe cases, conservative therapy may not help, and the condition may further worsen causing osteoarthritis of the first MTP joint. It can also result in deformities in the other toes.

Surgical Treatment: Surgical correction of the malformation in the metatarsal bone is performed. Soft tissue enlargements that may be seen in the ball of the foot can also be removed surgically.

Regenerative therapy: When conservative therapy is not successful in treating hallux valgus, the new option is Prolotherapy. Prolotherapy injections given in and around the painful areas help in healing the degenerative changes and promote new connective tissue growth. Patients can experience a drastic change in their ability to exercise and perform their activities of daily living.

Fractures: Malunion/Nonunion

Trauma to the bones in the feet and ankle can cause fractures. Sometimes these fractures may not heal in a proper fashion. If the fracture heals in a different position causing a deformity or shortening of the limb, it is known as a malunion. When the fracture fails to heal completely leading to pain and instability, it is called nonunion. Malunion or nonunion of fractures commonly occur due to problems with bone healing, improper bone alignment, or bone infections.

Fracture healing is dependent on two main factors: blood supply and soft-tissue health. Some of the causes for improper healing of fractures in the foot and ankle include diabetes, severe anemia, older age group, low vitamin D levels, hypothyroidism, poor nutrition, and use of tobacco (smoking). Proper immobilization is also a very important requirement for good fracture healing.

Symptoms: There may be a swelling in the fracture site. Patients may continue to experience pain at the fracture site even weeks or months after the trauma. There may be tenderness (pain on touching) in the area. Visible deformity of the bone may be present. There will be instability of the joints and the person will experience difficulty in bearing weight on the affected side.

Diagnosis: Gross deformities may be present, which help in the diagnosis of a malunion. A gap in the bone can be palpated in cases of nonunion of fractures. Imaging modalities such as X-ray, MRI, and CT scans play an important role in the diagnosis. Repeat imaging will allow the surgeon to follow the progress of fracture healing and identify nonunion and malunion of fractures. Nonunion of bone is diagnosed when there is no progress in bone healing even after several months.

Treatment: Conventional treatment for fracture nonunion or malunion is usually surgery. In the case of malunion, a cut or 'osteotomy' is performed near the original fracture site to correct the mal-alignment. An added fixation is applied to hold the bones in the correct position and aid faster healing. For nonunion fractures, the surgeon will take steps to restore the damaged bones and tissues around the fracture site. Bone grafting can be done to 'jump-start' the healing process. Here, the surgeon will harvest small pieces of bone from other areas in the body and transplant them at the nonunion site. These pieces have fresh bone cells that help in restoring the deficient bone. At times, bone substitutes also may be used. Internal or external fixation of the fracture site is required as well for proper bone healing.

Regenerative therapy: As we have seen, the treatment of nonunion fractures can be challenging for orthopedic surgeons. Moreover, there may be some patients who are not good candidates for surgical management of their nonunion fractures.

The use of biological agents to promote bone healing has been extensively studied in recent times. A few studies have provided level IV evidence (based on individual patient response) that the use of platelet-rich plasma (PrP) accelerated fracture healing. Basically, PrP mimics the role of a hematoma, which usually forms at a fracture site. Platelet cells in the hematoma enhance the healing process through various factors they release such as the epidermal growth factor and the vascular endothelial growth factor. PrP is said to augment fracture healing in the same way.

Chronic Pain At Healed Fracture Site

All of us know that a fractured bone in the foot or ankle will cause acute pain. But many a time, the healing process continues to be painful. In fact, a few people experience chronic pain at the fracture site even after complete healing. The pain that is experienced during the healing process is described as subacute pain. This pain results from the immobilization maintained for fracture healing. Inactivity of the affected part of the foot causes stiffness in the soft tissues around the injury site. There is also a weakening of the muscles in the area of the fracture.

Scarring and inflammation can occur in the soft tissues, and this can cause pain on moving the foot. Some people continue to experience chronic pain at the site of the trauma long after the fracture and the affected soft tissues have completely healed. This pain is usually a result of nerve damage or the formation of scar tissue. Sometimes there may be an aggravation of an underlying arthritic condition.

Symptoms: The patient complains of chronic pain at the site of a healed fracture.

Diagnosis: X-ray imaging is done to confirm fracture healing. MRI scan can help detect soft tissue inflammation in surrounding structures or arthritic changes in the joints.

Treatment: We have already looked at how acute pain associated with fractures in the foot and ankle may be treated. Subacute pain is treated mainly with physical therapy and exercises that can strengthen the weakened muscles and improve the range of movements.

Chronic pain is again treated with physical therapy and exercises. The patients may be prescribed pain relief medications. When chronic pain is not managed by these methods, it seriously affects the daily activities of the patients and their quality of life.

Regenerative therapy: As we have seen before, Prolotherapy is said to help in reducing chronic pain by accelerating the healing process of the underlying condition.

Retrocalcaneal Bursitis

This condition is also known as bursitis of the heel. A bursa is a fluid-filled sac. Bursae are present around all the large joints in our body. The function of the bursa is to act as a lubricant or a cushion over which the tendons can slide instead of directly moving on the underlying bone. The retrocalcaneal bursa is located behind the heel bone or the calcaneus. Excessive use of the ankle joint can result in irritation and inflammation of the bursa. The common activities that cause this condition are prolonged walking or jumping. Retrocalcaneal bursitis is commonly seen in athletes and ballet dancers. It can also be caused by wearing poorly fitting shoes.

Symptoms:

Pain present at the back of the heel that comes on with activities like running or jumping.
- The area is painful to touch as well.
- Swelling is present on the back of the heel.
- Standing on tiptoes can make the pain worse.
- Increased warmth may be present over the back of the heel. This is a sign of inflammation.

Diagnosis: A good evaluation of the back of the heel by your orthopedic surgeon will help in the diagnosis. Examination of the Achilles tendon, the calcaneal bone, and the bursa is made by the doctor. X-ray imaging can help in supporting the clinician's diagnosis of retrocalcaneal bursitis. MRI scanning will help detect the presence of inflammation.

Treatment:

Conservative Therapy: Treatment is mostly conservative.
- Resting the affected foot and ankle adequately.
- Keeping the foot in the elevated position.
- Applying an ice pack around the affected heel three to four times a day.
- Wearing custom-made shoes with wedges. They help to decrease heel stress.
- Taking anti-inflammatory medication.
- Physical therapy and gentle stretching exercises.
- Steroid injections given into the bursa in patients who do not respond to the other remedies.

Surgical Management: Very rarely in an unresolved case of bursitis, it may be necessary to perform a bursectomy—surgical removal of the bursa. Retrocalcaneal bursitis can be prevented by exercising the ankle joint and ensuring that there is good flexibility. Also, take care to wear proper fitting footwear. Make sure that your footwear is not too tight, and it provides good support to the arches of the foot.

Regenerative Therapy: Heel bursitis will resolve with conservative therapy when it is not an advanced or complicated condition. But patients suffer from chronic pain when they have heel bursitis complicated with other conditions like tendon tears.
Chronic calcaneal bursitis is difficult to manage and severely impacts the quality of life. PrP plus Prolotherapy has been used in managing these patients. It helps by augmenting tissue regeneration and healing.

Osteoarthritis of Foot and Ankle

As we have seen, arthritis of any joint involves inflammation in and around that particular joint. The same holds true for osteoarthritis of the foot and ankle joints as well. There are 28 bones and 33 joints in the foot.

The numerous bones and joints present in the foot and ankle allow for extensive flexibility and movement. Inflammation of these joints often results in pain, stiffness, and swelling. The more commonly affected joints in the foot will be where the ankle meets the shin bone (tibiotalar joint), the joints present between the heel bone and the midfoot bones, and the joint of the big toe and foot (first metatarsophalangeal joint).

In arthritis, there are progressive degenerative changes that occur in the joint with the destruction of the articular cartilages. As a result, the 'cushioning' effect is lost and the articulating bones rub against each other, leading to the wearing down of the bones. The damage can extend to the ligaments, tendons, and soft tissues present around the affected joints as well. There are some conditions that predispose to developing arthritis of the foot and ankle.

- Obesity
- Family history of osteoarthritis
- History of rheumatoid arthritis or gout
- Frequent injuries of the foot and ankle region

The ligaments around the ankle joint become weaker and lead to instability of the joint. As the affected bone tries to repair the damage, bone spurs can develop, which will add to the pain experienced.

Symptoms:
- Tenderness and pain will be experienced in the joint.
- You will experience difficulty in walking or moving your foot.

- The affected joints will be stiff.
- There may be a swelling present in the joint.
- Patients may experience increased pain and swelling on getting up in the morning or after prolonged sitting.
- In some patients, moving the foot will result in a grating or crackling sensation or noise.
- Vigorous activity, standing for a long time, and wearing high heels can cause exacerbation of the pain.

Diagnosis: The clinician will record a detailed history of the condition including details about when and where the pain started, and what are the factors that increase or decrease the pain. Gait analysis is performed, checking the stride of the patient and how they walk. X-ray imaging will reveal arthritic changes such as narrowing of joint space or the formation of bone spurs. Weight-bearing X-rays (taken in the standing position) are important in the diagnosis of foot and ankle arthritis as they point toward the severity of the disease and the presence of joint deformity. CT and MRI scans are useful for finding out the condition of the surrounding soft tissues. Lab tests are carried out to check for the presence of other arthritic conditions such as rheumatoid arthritis or gout.

Treatment: We have already seen that there is no cure for arthritis, but there are a number of ways in which one can manage or reduce the symptoms of pain and swelling and improve the mobility of the affected joints.

Conservative Management: Lifestyle changes can help in relieving pain and slowing down the progress of the disease.

Weight management: In the case of overweight patients, losing the excess weight helps by reducing the strain experienced by the feet and ankles.
Regular exercises. In osteoarthritis, exercise actually helps the

condition by strengthening the muscles and tendons around the affected joint. Walking daily is a good way to remain active, and it improves your health and general well-being as well. Swimming is another way of keeping fit, especially as it does not involve putting weight on the feet and ankles.

Physical therapy: Regular physiotherapy under expert guidance can go a long way in managing foot and ankle arthritis. The therapist can develop individualized exercise programs depending on the patient's needs and lifestyle. Stretching and strengthening exercises can be practiced.

Medications: Anti-inflammatory medications can help reduce the swelling in the foot and ankle. They help in controlling arthritic pain as well. In cases of severe pain, narcotic pain relievers are also used.

Steroid injections: In patients with severe pain and loss of mobility, steroid injections may be used in the affected ankle joint to reduce pain and swelling. The effects usually last only for a short while, though.

Foot supports: Braces, casts, custom-made footwear, sole inserts, and other assisted devices like walkers or canes might help minimize the pressure on the affected foot and decrease the pain.

Surgical Management: When the conservative methods fail to control the pain or improve mobility in a case of osteoarthritis of the foot and ankle, surgical treatment might be resorted to.

Arthroscopy and debridement: This procedure is useful mainly in the early stages of arthritis. This is usually a 'keyhole' procedure where small incisions are made on the sides of the affected ankle, or around the big toe if the first metatarsophalangeal joint is affected. The incisions are generally less than 1 cm in length and the surgeon visualizes the interior using a probe.

Concomitantly, bone spurs, loose cartilage, and inflamed synovial tissue are removed. In some patients, arthroscopy can result in increased arthritic deterioration of the joint.

Arthrodesis: Here, all the bones in the foot and ankle are fused completely such that it is one continuous bone, or maybe two. The idea is to decrease the pain by eliminating movement in the joint. Rods, plates, and screws are used for the fixation. There may be delayed wound healing in a few patients. This is an irreversible procedure and careful thought must be given before deciding to undergo this surgery.

Arthroplasty: This refers to ankle joint replacement surgery. The surgeon removes the damaged cartilage and bone in the ankle joint and replaces them with new metal or plastic joint implants to restore the joint function. A plastic spacer may be inserted between two surfaces of the bones. Arthroplasty helps improve pain and range of movements of the joint. However, it is said that ankle replacements usually last for about 10 years only.

Regenerative Therapy: Regenerative therapy can slow down the degenerative process in arthritis of the foot and ankle. PrP prolotherapy helps by decreasing pain and promoting healing in the affected joints. It can take away the need to undergo surgery or delay the requirement for surgical management considerably.

─────※─────

CASE STUDY 10

Santosh was a 42-year-old IT professional. He was around 5'11" tall, and slightly overweight. He was not definitely in the obese category. He was a brilliant student and had passed out from the Indian Institute of Technology (IIT) Madras.

He was an allrounder, excelling in his studies and in sports. During his student days, he had extensively played football and basketball. In the course of his sportsman days, he had experienced recurrent ankle sprains and injuries. He would not let these injuries hinder him in any way.

Even after sustaining an injury, he was famous for bulldozing his way through many matches by strapping his leg with a crepe bandage. He had completed many tournaments in this fashion without giving a second thought to his injuries. When the pain was a little intense, he would resort to taking anti-inflammatory medications.

Once the pain had resolved a bit, he would start playing again. Even when his student days were behind him, he continued to follow an active lifestyle. He was an active participant in all the activities organized by his friends like hiking and trekking. He continued to play basketball with a local team from his workplace whenever time permitted. He started noticing increasing instability in his left ankle a few years ago. It appeared like the left ankle was weak and prone to injury. He often sustained sprains in the left ankle, but would manage it just as he did in the old times—a few days' rest, strapping, and some pain-relieving medicines. However, the pain has now become increasingly frequent, and it does not settle down as before either. At the present time, he experiences pain in the left ankle with many of his daily activities, and any exertional or weight-bearing activity definitely incapacitates him.

He went for a consultation with an orthopedic surgeon. After examining him and evaluating his X-ray and MRI scan images, he was diagnosed to have multiple issues in his left ankle. Many of the ligaments in the ankle were injured and weak as a result of many years of neglect and improper treatment. He was found to have anterior talofibular (ATFL) and posterior talofibular (PTFL) ligament injuries. These injuries are more common among athletes. He had a complete tear of the ATFL, which is a Grade 3 injury. This explained the joint instability he experienced and why he was unable to bear weight on that joint.

The orthopedic surgeon advised that he undergo surgery to repair the tear. Another doctor told him that only isolated ATFL tears are successfully treated by surgery. Since he had other ligament involvement as well, surgery may not be successful. This confused him, and he was in a quandary as to his next move.

On the advice of a colleague, he visited another surgeon, who performed an arthroscopic debridement on the left ankle to reduce the pain. This arthroscopic washout procedure too was not successful in decreasing his pain.

This was when he came to us at ALLEVIATE. Our consultants carefully noted his medical history and performed a thorough physical examination. Soft tissue MRI scanning showed extensive changes and damage in the tendons around the left ankle joint. Along with the involvement of the ATFL AND PTFL, he was also diagnosed with peroneus tendonitis. This condition is also more commonly seen in sportsmen who take part in excessive weight-bearing activities like walking, running, and jumping. Concomitant Achilles tendon inflammation was also found to be present.

We explained to him exactly what had happened to his ankle joint over the many years of neglect. Multiple ligaments had endured repeated trauma and the degenerative process had started in these.

At Alleviate, he was treated with image-guided PrP plus extensive Prolotherapy. We clearly told him that the process of recovery would be long and take time, because the damage to the ankle had also been sustained over a long period. He underwent multiple sessions of image-guided Prolotherapy.

Since a multidisciplinary approach fetches the best results, he also was advised about proper exercise and diet. He ensured that he was regular for his physiotherapy sessions and followed the diet chart prescribed for him by our nutritionist. He was able to reduce his weight, which contributed to his general health and wellbeing. He soon began to feel so much better. He never expected that his pain and symptoms would improve to this extent.

CASE STUDY 11

Latha was a 52-year-old chemistry professor working in a well-known women's college in Bangalore. She was married and had two children. She had been in the teaching profession for many years. She resided in the suburbs and faced a long commute by public transport to and from her workplace every day. She had been experiencing pain in her feet for many years, which she did not take seriously. She attributed the pain to her long hours of standing during travel by bus and also standing in the college while teaching. She told herself that it was bound to happen. Her life was so busy that she hardly found time for herself. Whenever she had pain, she would apply some local pain gel or ask one of her children to massage her feet. On a few rare occasions when she had enough time, she would soak her legs in warm water before going to bed and feel a bit relaxed.

After a few years, the pain appeared to be getting more severe and she started taking some anti-inflammatory and pain-relieving medicines for the same. There would be some temporary relief, but the pain in both her feet would recur. She went for an orthopedic consultation. The surgeon diagnosed her to have plantar fasciitis and suggested that she receive steroid injections.

She agreed and took the treatment which was given blind and not under image guidance. She experienced relief from the pain, which lasted for a couple of years. Once again, she started having pain in her feet and went for repeat treatment with steroid injections. After two such attempts with steroid injection therapy, she did not get complete relief from the pain. She came to us at this stage. At Alleviate, we evaluated her thoroughly. We found that she was slightly overweight and was using poorly fitting footwear as well. She gave a history of experiencing heel pain as soon as she got out of bed in the morning and took her first steps.

The pain would decrease as she got on with her household activities. She also noticed increased pain when she got up after sitting for a long time.

We confirmed that she had plantar fasciitis and explained the condition to her. We stressed the importance of other lifestyle changes she would have to make as well. She underwent therapy with image-guided PrP injections to the plantar fascia. She attended multiple sessions of therapy and also underwent about two weeks of physiotherapy. She was given advice on choosing suitable footwear and the nutritionist gave her a diet chart to follow. She experienced marked relief from the pain and was able to return to her routine activities without any discomfort.

As you can see from these cases, foot and ankle conditions are very much neglected by people because they think they are not important or serious. Another factor is that most people are not aware of the serious consequences that can arise when foot and ankle conditions are neglected. People care more for their cars than they do for their feet. As noted at the beginning of this chapter your feet are your 'wheels' that are responsible for moving you from one place to another. They bear the whole weight of your body as well. They are entitled to proper care and maintenance.

How can you care for your feet?

- Never ignore foot pain
- Keep your feet clean and dry.
- Moisturize your feet and keep your toenails cut neatly.
- Wear proper fitting and comfortable footwear. Do not sacrifice comfort and safety for style. Buy footwear only in the evenings to ensure a proper fit.
- Maintain the ideal body weight.

Another reason for people neglecting their painful foot conditions is unawareness about the new management methods that they can avail. Regenerative therapy is one such method.

Regenerative therapy like Prolotherapy helps to rebuild damaged tissues. It promotes new tissue growth in degenerative conditions and helps to relieve pain significantly. If you are someone suffering from longstanding pain in the feet, or you know someone who does, make a visit to Alleviate and we will guide you.

Precepts and Precautions

1. Your feet help you move around; they are your 'wheels.'
2. Make foot care a part of your daily routine.
3. Do not consider foot pain as an inevitable part of aging.
4. Prevention is better than cure—the adage holds true for conditions of the feet as well.
5. Any pain in the feet should be investigated promptly.
6. Foot problems may occur due to systemic causes (rheumatoid arthritis, diabetes) or localized causes (trauma, tendonitis).
7. Loss of mobility can have a major impact on your life: loss of independence, inability to carry out normal roles, loss of confidence, etc.
8. Neglected foot problems can eventually affect the knee, hip, and spine as well.
9. Fit the shoe to the feet, not the other way around

7

INTERVENTIONAL PAIN MANAGEMENT

You don't have to live with it

To relieve another's pain is the highest calling one can have. Life with any chronic pain can be quite debilitating. What exactly do we mean by chronic pain? Any pain that has been present for a period longer than six months is usually termed chronic pain. 'Pain' usually heralds the presence of an injury or a disease. We are aware of this. But many times, even after the injury or the disease has been cured, people continue to suffer from pain. What can be done in such a scenario?

If you are a person interested in gardening or a lover of plants, you would know all the requirements for a healthy plant or tree. Let us assume you have a favorite plant in your garden. It is a flowering plant and you have been enjoying its fragrant blooms for some time now. One day as you are strolling in your garden you notice that your plant does not appear as perky as it used to. The leaves appear to be drooping and there are only a few blooms. You water your plant and believe it will recover. However, a few days later you notice that your favorite flowering plant has not recovered, rather it has worsened.

The plant appears quite leafless. Many leaves have dried and there are absolutely no blooms for you to enjoy.

What will your first reaction be? Will you tell yourself, "Oh, well! That's your fate." Or will you get your gardener to immediately chop it down? No! You will not do either of these. Your first reaction will be to find out what is causing your plant to be 'ill.' Then you will see how it can be cured. You will ask someone who is an expert in gardening or a professional horticulturist about the symptoms shown by your plant. You will check if your plant is getting enough sunlight. Maybe there is some fungal infection. You will find out what spray or insecticide you can use to remedy the situation. Sometimes the plant may not be getting the required nutrients to bloom. The soil quality may not be up to the mark. In such a case, you will change the soil and add more fertilizers as needed.

Pruning or removing the plant will only be the last step you will take. Only when none of the other measures help in saving the plant will you resort to such a drastic step. The same is true for the body as well. When we have a physical ailment or disease, we do not immediately go for drastic measures. We start with simple therapies. But most important before beginning any therapy is to know what the problem is. After we are aware of the exact disease or condition, we look for the right treatment. As we saw in the previous chapters, the initial therapy would be conservative management, which includes medicines, diet, physical exercise, and other supportive measures. Next in line comes interventional management. This basically means that the doctor or clinician is providing treatment through some intervention like injections or intravenous fluids.

This is not a drastic method of treatment like surgical therapy, which is the last resort. Interventional management has a role to play in Pain therapy as well, especially, in patients with chronic pain. So, what exactly is Interventional Pain management. The American Society of Interventional Pain Physicians (ASIPP) defines interventional pain management this way:

Interventional pain management is a discipline of medicine devoted to the diagnosis and treatment of pain-related disorders.

Here the aim is to relieve, reduce, or manage pain in such a way as to improve the functionality and the quality of a patient's life using minimally invasive procedures that are specifically targeted for the particular patient's condition. Let us see the various methods of interventional pain management that are being used in the treatment of chronic pain.

1. Myofascial Trigger Point Injections:

Trigger point injections are used by doctors to treat chronic pain in the muscles. The myofascial trigger points consist of highly sensitive muscle fibers in tight bands. Injections are given directly to the affected muscle fibers. The drugs that may be used are as follows:

(a) Local anesthetics: Local anesthetics such as lidocaine can be injected, which reduces pain by blocking the pain receptors in the affected muscle.

(b) Corticosteroids: Injection of steroids into the muscles and connective tissues can help reduce inflammation and swelling. This in turn will decrease the irritability of neighboring nerve endings, thereby reducing pain.

(c) Botulinum Toxin A: This is used in some specific conditions. It interferes with the nerve signaling pathway and thereby reduces muscle contractions.

Uses of trigger point injections:
- Myofascial Pain Syndrome
- Fibromyalgia
- Headaches (migraine, tension headaches)

Trigger point injections can cause some side effects such as pain or numbness around the injection site, discoloration at the injection site, and bleeding. In rare cases, muscle damage can occur. Pain and swelling around the injection site usually disappear after a few hours. People have reported significant pain relief following trigger point therapy, either immediately or after several days or weeks.

However, a few patients have reported no relief from their pain.

2. Anti-inflammatory Injections (Spine):

Powerful anti-inflammatory injections are sometimes injected directly into the epidural space in the spinal cord. Steroid injections are the common option. They are used to relieve chronic back pain or leg pain. They reduce pain by reducing inflammation that is present around the nerves. This helps in improving the mobility and function of the limbs. The pain relief may be temporary, lasting from a few weeks to one year. Repeat injections may be necessary.

Some of the conditions where epidural steroid injections are used are as follows:

- Disc herniation
- Degenerative disc disease
- Spinal canal stenosis

Patients can experience some side effects following steroid injections in the spine, such as pain in the injection site, nausea, headache, and dizziness. These side effects usually resolve in a few hours. Very rarely serious complications such as stroke or spinal cord damage can occur. That is why it is very important that only experienced persons should administer epidural steroid injections. This treatment is administered by spine surgeons, neurologists, pain management specialists, anesthesiologists, or radiologists. It is performed under image guidance. Fluoroscopic X-ray is used to locate the exact vertebral level for injecting the steroid and live images can be seen on a computer screen. A local anesthetic is first injected into the skin to numb the area before the steroid is administered into the epidural space. This therapy is mainly used in treating conditions relating to the lumbar spine, such as sciatica.

Steroid injections to the spine are contra-indicated in patients who have infections anywhere in the body, bleeding disorders, or cancer. The patient is advised to take some precautions following the procedure.

Driving and strenuous physical activities are not recommended for one day. Ice packs may be used intermittently for localized pain at the injection site. Additional epidural steroid injections are given only in certain conditions. If the first injection was successful in reducing the pain by 50 percent or more, and the effect lasted for a month or more, then an additional injection may be given when the effect of the first wears off. It is not recommended to give more than three epidural steroid injections in a year.

3. Radiofrequency (RF) Procedures:

Radiofrequency ablation is a minimally invasive procedure that uses heat to decrease or remove pain. Basically, the nerve fibers carrying pain signals are destroyed in this procedure. It is mainly used to treat painful conditions in the spine. It is also said to provide good pain relief for those suffering from chronic pain in the face, neck, or shoulder regions. The procedure is performed under image guidance by someone who is trained in the technic, such as a radiologist, neurologist, anesthesiologist, or surgeon. It is usually an outpatient procedure and the patient can go home the same day. It is contraindicated in those who have infections or bleeding disorders.

In this procedure, RF current is passed through a hollow needle to cause small precise burns that are called lesions. A portion of the nerve causing pain is thereby destroyed and the pain pathway is interrupted. Patients may experience some local pain following the procedure for a few days. The effect of RF ablation is said to last from 9 months to 2 years. If the pain recurs due to regrowth of the nerves, the procedure may be repeated. A few side effects that may occur are a temporary increase in nerve pain, localized numbness, neuroma, infection at the site, allergic reaction, etc.

RF ablation has been reported to be very effective in reducing pain in shoulder joint conditions such as osteoarthritis or rotator cuff injuries. Being a freely movable joint, the shoulder is prone to a lot of injuries. Sports injuries are also common in the shoulder joint. Pain resulting from all these can be helped by RF ablation.

4. Spinal Cord Stimulation:

Spinal cord stimulation is a new method to control chronic pain, especially in those who suffer from intractable back, leg, or arm pain. Here a small device is used to mask the pain signals before they reach the brain. The device is placed surgically under the skin and sends mild electric impulses to the spinal cord. These electric impulses can modify and mask the pain signals being carried to the brain. Here the source of pain is not removed, rather the perception of pain by the brain is changed. It is recommended for patients who have chronic debilitating pain lasting for more than three months in the lower back, leg, or arm.

Spinal cord stimulation can be used in the following conditions:
- Chronic leg pain (sciatica)
- Diabetic neuropathy
- Failed back surgery
- Arachnoiditis (inflammation of the lining of the spinal nerves)
- Stump pain following amputations
- Peripheral vascular disease
- Multiple sclerosis
- Spinal cord injury

The procedure can be performed by neurosurgeons or doctors who specialize in pain management. First, a temporary trial is undertaken to see if the method is successful in decreasing pain. If it is, then the device is placed under the skin. The procedure is performed under image guidance. A small skin incision is made in the middle of the back under local anesthesia and the vertebral column is exposed. A portion of the bony arch of the vertebra is removed to make space and the leads are positioned and secured with sutures. The leads do not directly touch the spinal cord. The lead wires are then passed under the skin up to the buttocks where the generator device is placed.

You will have to follow some recommendations following the procedure for about six to eight weeks, such as not lifting any heavy objects, not doing strenuous activity, no alcohol intake, and no driving.

The procedure can have some side effects like an epidural hematoma, hemorrhage, or infection, cerebrospinal fluid leak, lead migration, battery failure, allergic response, or undesirable discharges. Studies have reported spinal cord stimulation to provide good pain relief in 50 to 80 percent of patients. This is a reversible procedure and the leads and generator can be removed if required.

5. **Endoscopic spine surgery:** This is a surgical procedure where very small incisions (less than 1 inch) are made and an endoscope is used to visualize the disc and the inside of the spinal canal. Tubular structures are used to gain access to the surgical field. It is an advanced minimally invasive spine surgery. When compared to conventional spine surgery techniques, the patients experience lesser recurring pain and a quicker recovery time.

   Endoscopic spine procedures are used to manage the following conditions:

   - Disc herniation
   - Spinal canal stenosis
   - Fusion surgeries

Endoscopic spine surgeries are performed while treating adolescents or athletes for lumbar disc herniation where less tissue trauma, cosmesis, and early recovery of function are desirable. Endoscopic spine procedures can help relieve back pain without the complications and prolonged recovery time seen with conventional surgical treatment.

Some of the surgeries performed by this technique are listed below:

- Endoscopic discectomy. It is the least invasive procedure to treat herniated, protruding, or bulging discs.

- Endoscopic spine decompression. Tissue causing pressure on the spinal cord can be removed endoscopically.
- Endoscopic lumbar fusion. Following a complete endoscopic discectomy, bone grafts are inserted in the intervertebral space using a small tube.
- Endoscopic disc debridement. Discitis caused by bacteria can be debrided by this method. Used to relieve pressure from a herniated disc, scar tissue, or bone spurs.
- Endoscopic rhizotomy. Used to treat patients with chronic low back pain and muscle spasms.
- Endoscopic laminotomy. This procedure is performed in patients with lumbar stenosis who do not respond to conventional treatment.

Endoscopic spine surgery has many advantages. Smaller incisions are used, which means there is less trauma to the skin, muscle, and soft tissues. This results in lesser blood loss and faster healing. Post-operative recovery time is reduced as well. It can be a day procedure and the patient can go home the same day.

However, as it is a specialized procedure, skilled spine surgeons are required to perform it. The procedure can cost more than conventional spine surgery because specialized instruments are required.

6. Nerve blocks:

Nerve blocks are used for treating chronic pain that cannot be managed by pain medications or other therapies. They relieve pain by interrupting the pain signals that are being sent to the brain. Usually, a substance such as phenol or alcohol is injected around a nerve plexus. Alcohol blocks give pain relief for a longer time. Nerve blocks may be classified as surgical and non-surgical. In surgical nerve blocks, the nerves in an extended area may be blocked as in sympathetic blockade or splanchnic plexus block. Non-surgical nerve blocks include epidural and spinal anesthesia procedures.

These are some of the chronic pain common conditions for which nerve blocks are used:

- Cancer-related pain
- Arthritis pain
- Severe facial pain (trigeminal neuralgia)
- Low back pain
- Headaches (migraine and occipital neuralgia)
- Chronic regional pain syndrome

Sometimes nerve blocks are used to find out the cause of chronic pain as well. Celiac plexus block is used to treat severe pain caused by pancreatic cancer or other abdominal cancers. The procedure is performed under image guidance to visualize the proper positioning of the needle. Either a local anesthetic or alcohol is injected into the celiac plexus. Another nerve plexus block that is used in cancer pain is the splanchnic plexus block.

There are many benefits from a nerve block. Patients experience significant relief from pain following a nerve block procedure. It helps people suffering from chronic pain to lead a better quality of life, enabling them to work or perform their daily activities without pain. There may be a few rare side effects like bleeding at the injection site or infection. People who already have an infection, bleeding disorders, or prior nerve conditions should not be given nerve blocks. What are some of the conditions that can benefit from interventional pain management?

CASE STUDY 12

Sathish was a 56-year-old business executive. He was a very health-conscious person with a happy-go-lucky nature.

About eight years ago, he had to visit a dentist for treatment of an impacted tooth in the upper jaw on the left side. The dentist diagnosed the condition as an impacted third molar and advised extraction. Accordingly, he underwent extraction of the problematic tooth.

Following the procedure, Sathish started experiencing what he termed as weird symptoms of intense pain and numbness on the left side of his face. Initially, he tried to ignore them as he thought they were sequelae of the local anesthetic that was used for the tooth extraction. The pain would come on suddenly and last only for about half a minute. However, the symptom did not disappear even after many months. He went back to the dentist who advised root canal treatment saying that the pain was caused by a deep-seated infection. However, this did not cure him of the pain. The onset of pain was unpredictable. There would be weeks and even months when he was pain-free leading him to think that he was cured. But the pain kept returning. Anything could trigger the burning pain he felt. Sometimes just wiping his face on a towel after washing would trigger an episode. At other times the pain would come on suddenly while chewing food. Once when he was on a seaside holiday, he experienced sudden sharp shooting pain just as he was walking along the beach and a cool breeze brushed his face.

There was no telling when the pain would appear. As time went by the pain increased in intensity and duration too. The painful episodes lasted longer now. This made him very anxious and his family noticed that his whole personality was changing. From a happy-go-lucky person, he now became a worried and short-tempered one. He was constantly dreading the arrival of the facial pain.

He consulted a general physician who prescribed some pain killers. These medications did not help him in any way. It was at this stage that he visited us at Alleviate. He came to us on the recommendation of a colleague whose relative had been treated at our clinic successfully for a knee joint problem. After going through his medical and dental history, and ruling out any dental pathology based on dental x-ray imaging, we were able to diagnose his condition as Trigeminal Neuralgia. Once the diagnosis was made, we treated him with image-guided radiofrequency ablation. Following this procedure, the patient experienced relief from the pain. He was relieved of the suffering that he had undergone for eight long years.

Let us learn more about Trigeminal Neuralgia

Trigeminal Neuralgia

Trigeminal neuralgia can be described as pain arising in the trigeminal nerve. It usually occurs only on one side, but there are some patients who are affected on both sides. The trigeminal nerve is a cranial nerve that carries sensation from the face to the brain. It has three branches that enervate the upper, middle, and lower portions of the face. Depending on which branch is affected, the respective area of the face will experience the pain. Most often, the pain occurs in the lower part of the face. The condition often occurs spontaneously, but sometimes it can follow a dental procedure or any trauma to the face. The main cause is said to be vascular compression: a blood vessel pressing on the trigeminal nerve.

The pulsations of the artery can cause the myelin sheath of the nerve to be worn away leading to exposure and increased sensitivity. Another condition associated with trigeminal neuralgia is multiple sclerosis, where there is deterioration of the myelin sheath of the trigeminal nerve. Injuries to the trigeminal nerve following dental procedures can also cause this condition. In trigeminal neuralgia, even gentle stimulation of the face like washing with water, wiping dry with a towel, a soft breeze, or brushing teeth can trigger severe pain along the nerve.

Initially, the pain may be like a flash lasting only a few seconds. However, it can progressively last for longer periods of time, up to many minutes.

Symptoms

Pain: This is the predominant symptom of this condition. The type of pain can vary—It can be sudden stabbing or shooting pain in the cheek, or it can be a constant burning sensation. The pain can last from a few seconds to several minutes. The pain is felt mainly in areas supplied by this nerve including the cheek, jaw, teeth, gums, or lips. Less often, the pain may involve the eye or the forehead.

Pain-free intervals: The condition is generally progressive, but the patients can experience periods of relief from the pain. In the initial stages, there may even be a gap of a year or so between episodes. However, the frequency and intensity of the attacks increase over time.

Anxiety: The debilitating effect of this condition is the constant worry and anxiety about the pain. The quality of life of the patient is severely affected. Some people avoid social engagements because of the fear of an attack of pain.

It leads to depression or even suicidal thoughts in some patients who have severe painful episodes of trigeminal neuralgia. The unpredictability of the occurrence of pain is one of the main causes of anxiety in these people.

Diagnosis:

1.   Comprehensive medical history including details about the onset of pain and triggering factors. Other disorders that cause facial pain such as post-herpetic neuralgia and temporomandibular joint disorders should be ruled out.
2.   Thorough physical examination to rule out other causes of facial pain like dental caries.
3.   Imaging studies such as CAT scan and high-resolution MRI of the trigeminal nerve and the surrounding areas to check for a tumor or a blood vessel abnormality.

Management:

1. Medications: Seizure-controlling medications such as Carbamazepine and Gabapentin are used in some patients to control the episodes of pain.
2. Nerve Blocks: Steroids or other medications are sometimes injected into different sections of the nerve to reduce the pain. This can provide temporary pain relief for patients with trigeminal neuralgia.
3. Surgery: There are some surgical options that doctors use in patients with intractable pain, not amenable to medical treatment. These are Rhizotomy, MVD, and Stereotactic radiosurgery. Surgery in this area is a delicate and precise procedure and must be attempted only by experienced neurosurgeons.
4. Radiofrequency Ablation: Ablation basically means removing or destroying something. In radiofrequency ablation high-frequency heat is directed at the targeted areas of the body. In trigeminal neuralgia, the target is the trigeminal nerve. The procedure is performed under image guidance and the ability of the nerve to transmit pain signals to the brain is destroyed.

CASE STUDY 13

Serita was a 38-year-old housewife who was diagnosed with an abdominal malignancy in the tertiary stage. She was found to have cancer of the stomach with multiple secondaries. Her doctors had not given a good prognosis based on the extent of the spread of the disease. However, she was in terrible, continuous pain when she was brought to our clinic.

The family members were aware of the poor prognosis of one or two years given by the doctor, but they were very disturbed by the fact that she was in severe pain. They were not able to witness her intolerable pain and suffering. When she was brought to Alleviate, we assessed her condition and found that she had not been prescribed the correct dosage of pain regulatory medications, which was contributing to her severe distress and pain.

She was treated with celiac plexus block and splanchnic block. These procedures are being increasingly used in the management of chronic pain in patients suffering from malignancies of the pancreas, liver, gall bladder, omentum, mesentery, and the alimentary tract—stomach to the transverse colon. We also managed her morphine requirement so that she was getting an adequate dosage of morphine. Her relatives came to see us about 10 months later and on enquiring they informed us that Serita had passed away about three months before. They were, however, very grateful to us that her last months were spent pain-free and in comfort. Interventional pain management can help in palliative pain therapy in such patients.

Chronic Pain in Malignancy[4]
Chronic pain in cancer patients can occur due to these reasons:
  (a) Pain caused by the primary cancer
  (b) Pain caused by the metastases
  (c) Pain caused by the treatment of cancer (post-cancer)
Etiology: Pain in cancer can arise from the tumor pressing on adjacent structures like bones, nerves, or soft tissues. The severity of pain depends on the type of cancer, location of the tumor, stage of the disease, and the presence of any nerve damage, either from cancer per se or from the treatment like surgery or radiation therapy.

---

[4]https://www.cancerresearchuk.org/about-cancer/coping/physically/cancer-and-pain-control/treating-pain

There are other more intangible factors that can have an effect on the pain perceived by cancer patients: fear anxiety, depression, or lack of sleep. Chronic pain in cancer can seriously affect the quality of life. It can make it hard for the person to perform their daily activities like bathing, shopping, cooking, and eating. One of the mainstays in cancer pain therapy is the use of painkillers They may be classified as opioid or non-opioid medications. However, some patients may be reluctant to take pain killers for various reasons such as fear of side effects or fear of addiction, in the case of narcotic medications. Some of the narcotic pain killers can also cause increased drowsiness and patients may be afraid of the drowsy feeling. Some patients equate the taking of painkillers to giving up the fight against cancer. This is not true. Pain medications are an aid to help you in your fight against cancer. It is important to talk about your pain and inform your caregivers and doctors as only then can they prescribe the right medication for you.

Management Of Cancer Pain

Managing cancer pain requires a multidisciplinary approach. At the first level, your doctor will be assessing you to find out more about your pain and then they will guide you to the right therapy that can provide relief. Let us see the various people who can help patients with chronic cancer pain.

1. You, the patient: It is important that you tell your doctor or your relatives about your pain. Sometimes patients tend to keep the pain to themselves in the misguided notion of not wanting to trouble anyone further. But you must understand that being in constant pain can make you feel very stressed and emotional. This can in turn affect your relationships. In the long run, it is better to get help for the pain. It will also help you cope better with any ongoing cancer treatments.

2. Palliative care doctors and nurses: They play a major role in pain management for cancer patients. You can see them at

the hospital or some even make home visits. They help in regulating the dosage of pain medications and also help in many other ways. It is important to take their support.

3. Anesthetists: They are very good at treating pain and can prescribe the best drug for pain control for each patient. Sometimes in cases of advanced disease, the cancer pain is intractable and does not respond to pain medications. In these situations, anesthetists can help by giving local anesthetic injections or performing nerve blocks.

4. Occupational therapists and physiotherapists: They provide good supportive treatment for cancer patients. Occupational therapists can give recommendations about how your day-to-day life can be made easier with proper equipment. Physiotherapists can provide massages and gentle exercises that can help you feel more relaxed.

5. Psychologists and counselors: They are an important part of the team for palliative relief of pain. They can help the patient to emotionally cope with the pain of cancer.

The various modes used for the treatment of cancer also aid in reducing the pain by reducing the bulk of a tumor or shrinking a tumor.

Let us see what the options are.

1. Chemotherapy or targeted drugs: These are medications that destroy the cancer cells and stop them from growing. They help in shrinking the tumor, thereby relieving pressure effects on nearby structures that might be causing pain.

2. Hormone therapy: Some cancers respond to hormone treatments that can slow or stop the growth of the tumors.

3. Radiotherapy: Radiation treatment to the targeted area can cause DNA damage in the cancer cells and destroy them. This can help reduce pain in certain cancers that involve the bone, etc.

4. Radiofrequency (RF) ablation: Heat from radio waves is used to kill cancer cells. This method is especially of use in patients for whom surgery is contraindicated.

5. Surgery: When there is a large tumor, a surgical procedure called debulking is performed to decrease pressure effects.

6. Nerve blocks: Injection of local anesthetics with steroids into the celiac nerve plexus can provide relief to patients with abdominal cancers.

There are several other conditions where interventional pain therapy can help. They are predominantly used in the management of various conditions affecting the muscles and the skeletal system (bones) as we saw in the previous chapters. If you are suffering from chronic pain due to any cause, which has not been relieved by medications.

If you do not want to undergo drastic surgical procedures or you are medically unfit for surgery, then the abovementioned interventional pain management techniques can definitely bring a ray of hope. Consider visiting a pain management specialist or visit us at Alleviate. We will do a complete assessment of your condition and see how best we can help you. We use the multidisciplinary approach and our doctors, physiotherapists, nutritionists, and counselors work together to provide a solution.

Precepts and Precautions

1. You do not have to live with chronic pain.
2. Get yourself checked and find out the reason for the pain.
3. Once you know the diagnosis, discuss the various options available for pain relief.
4. Interventional pain therapies help you have a better quality of life.
5. Interventional pain therapies are not addictive, rather they help you function better.

6. Patients with trigeminal neuralgia benefit greatly from RF ablation.

7. Pain caused by metastatic cancer can be controlled by various nerve blocks

8

THE REGENERATIVE REVOLUTION

"Take care of your body. It's the only place you have to live."
– Jim Rohn

In this chapter, I want to talk about regenerative medicine. The term may be new to you. You can call it futuristic medicine.

Our human body can be described as a wonderfully complex machine. A complex machine has multiple moving parts that are required to work in tandem for the machine to function in an optimal way. In the same way, the body too can be described as having numerous different parts that need to function correctly and smoothly for a healthy life. Our body supports us through all our days. The musculoskeletal system plays the main role in the movements of our body. It helps us move, walk, eat, run, work, and much more. The various components that make up the musculoskeletal system include bones, muscles, and ligaments. The joints in our body help us to be flexible and agile. Different joints perform different actions. For instance, the knee joint helps you in bending and stretching, whereas the hip joint allows the movements of bending, twisting, and turning.

The feet bear the entire weight of one's body. But for the body to move and function efficiently and effectively, it is necessary that all the various structures are in good form and maintained properly. You will remember how we talked about the importance of maintenance with regard to your car or machine

We need to give the same care to our body that we would give to a machine that we own like an air conditioner or a car. These machines too have numerous moving parts that are held together by various nuts, bolts, and levers. When new, your machine would perform effortlessly and efficiently. However, after some years of use, the various components in the machine would start showing signs of wear and tear. The machine may start to rust or there may be some loosening of the various nuts and bolts. The efficiency of the machine will come down. The said machine will start displaying signs of 'distress': the speed would decrease, noises may come from the machine, or it may not run as fast as it used to.

In such a situation, we usually immediately look into the matter to rectify it. We check to see if the machine needs a lubricant or oiling. Or maybe it needs the tightening of some loose nut or bolt. When we do not correct the problem immediately in a machine with multiple moving parts, the other parts start taking up the strain. This leads to their getting damaged as well. In the same way, our human bodies too can get worn down as we age and show signs of distress. And as we saw in the previous chapters, maintenance is mandatory to keep our bodies functioning smoothly.

Neglecting any disease or pain in the body anywhere is sure to lead to bigger problems later. For example, while talking about disc conditions in the spine, we see that the problem begins with the involvement of the disc at one level, but soon with neglect, the adjoining discs start bearing the strain, leading to degenerative changes in them as well.

This is true in degenerative conditions of the knee joint also, such as osteoarthritis. It initially affects the cartilage in the joint, but slowly as the condition progresses, it involves the collateral ligaments, which bear the brunt, and the quadriceps tendon, which also gets under heavy strain. This eventually leads to soft tissue imbalance.

What exactly is Regenerative Medicine? We are all aware that our body has the innate ability to heal itself up to a certain point. Regenerative medicine can be explained as therapy that helps to regrow or repair damaged or diseased tissues in the body by stimulating the body's own healing and repair mechanisms. Basically, we are trying to reproduce or trigger the inherent natural healing capability of the body.

Although at present, this branch of medicine is still in its infancy, it is promising to be a big part of medical practice in the coming days. We are the harbingers of this revolutionary step in managing chronic pain and our aim is to create awareness of these new methods of treatment among the people. We are taking the first step toward integrating regenerative therapies with mainstream treatment methods and bringing them into effective clinical practice. These new methods are particularly effective in the treatment of degenerative musculoskeletal conditions.

Hence, in simple terms, regenerative therapy can be described as a method of ensuring regular upkeep, service, and maintenance of our body. Regenerative medicine plays a huge role in bringing about a better quality of life to patients with degenerative conditions by reducing the symptoms and the pain associated with their disease.

Worldwide, a plethora of regenerative methods of treatment are being researched and some are under trial as well. However, in this chapter, I want to highlight three of these methods that have shown promising results and are currently available in our country.

Platelet-Rich Plasma Therapy

Platelet-rich plasma (PrP) therapy is one of the regenerative treatments that is coming to be used increasingly. Here, the natural growth factors present in our body are utilized to promote healing of the affected tissues.

Let us learn more about this procedure. Blood constitutes two main components: cells and plasma. The cells present in the blood are the red blood cells, white blood cells, and platelets. We all know that platelets are an important part of the clotting mechanism in our bodies. However, they also play a major role in bringing about healing in the body through various growth factors.

Plasma is the liquid portion of the blood. It is mainly constituted of water and proteins and helps in circulating the various cells throughout the body. Platelets while circulating in the body are in an inactivated state. An injury to the tissues can activate them, and they then congregate at the area of damage and release the various growth factors that promote healing and repair.

PrP is a concentrated preparation of the patient's own platelets. This is done by first taking a small quantity (30 to 50 ml) of blood from the patient and then centrifuging it. The heavier cells like red blood cells settle at the bottom of the tube and the plasma with the lighter cells, such as the platelets, rises to the top. This plasma with a high concentration of platelets is PrP. An activating factor is now added to these platelets and then they are injected directly into the diseased or damaged tissue that requires healing. The procedure is performed under image guidance. PrP is said to contain about five to six times the number of platelets that the normal whole blood has.

These platelets then release various growth factors that promote healing by increasing the number of new healthy cells in that part of the body. Some of the growth factors present in PrP are platelet-derived growth factor, vascular endothelial growth factor, epidermal growth factor, fibroblast growth factor, etc.

Uses of PrP: PrP is used in the management of tendon injuries, osteoarthritis, or other acute sports injuries. It is indicated in conditions where healing is not complete and the patient continues to be in pain. PrP is also used to promote healing following surgery for a rotator cuff tendon tear in the shoulder or an anterior cruciate ligament tear in the knee joint. PrP promotes healing and therefore it can reduce the need for pain medications in patients with chronic pain.

Benefits of PrP: It is a natural solution with the use of the patient's own blood. The process is simple and minimally invasive. The healing process is quickened. There are almost no side effects or allergic reactions. The rare side effects from this procedure would be pain at the injection site or infection.

Prolotherapy

Prolotherapy is otherwise known as proliferation therapy or regenerative injection therapy and can be described as maintenance therapy for painful or degenerative conditions. It can be compared to taking your car for servicing every six months or so. Prolotherapy is now being used to treat painful conditions of the musculoskeletal system. In this procedure, a natural irritant substance is injected into the soft tissue or the tendon of the affected joint. The irritant substance triggers the body's healing response. Prolotherapy is commonly being used to treat conditions affecting the knees, hips, shoulders, and back.

How is prolotherapy done? It involves the injecting of a sugar or saline solution into the affected ligament and tendon attachments. Dextrose solution combined with a local anesthetic is what is commonly used. When the body recognizes these as irritants, it mounts an immune response. The cells and chemicals required for healing move to the area and the natural healing process of the body gets started off. The exact mechanism of how prolotherapy works is not clear, but the basic underlying mechanism is the inflammatory response of the body. This inflammation promotes healing and results in the enlargement and strengthening of the damaged ligaments, tendons, and other structures.

Uses of Prolotherapy: Prolotherapy may be given to patients suffering from chronic low back pain, osteoarthritis, tendon injuries, or sports injuries. It is not recommended for use in patients who are suffering from cellulitis or septic arthritis.

Benefits of Prolotherapy: It brings about the healing of damaged ligaments and tendons. You can avoid the use of painkillers, which have harmful side effects. It is a natural treatment and no major side effects have been reported. Some of the mild effects of prolotherapy include pain at the site of injection or bleeding. There may be very rare cases of allergic reactions or infection.

Prolotherapy is usually given under image guidance and the procedure must be performed only by a trained person. Multiple sessions (three to five) are required for effective therapy.

Stem Cell Therapy

Stem cell therapy is a regenerative treatment that uses stem cells to repair diseased or injured tissue in the body. What do we mean by stem cells?

Stem cells are the first line of cells from which all other cell types originate. When stem cells divide, they can either become new daughter stem cells, or they can differentiate into specialized cells, such as red blood cells, cardiac muscle cells, and bone cells. Only stem cells have the ability to generate new cell types. So, this makes them very special.

Extensive research is being undertaken to see how stem cells can be used to generate healthy cells and replace diseased cells. Most often in adults, stem cells are harvested from the bone marrow.

Stem cell therapy has not yet been used in a big way in India, although It is being used in the West. There is a strong push toward making it a mainstream regenerative treatment method with increased awareness. PrP and Prolotherapy are the main regenerative therapies that are being used in our country. Numerous patients have benefitted from these therapies. Moreover, these remedies are rather safe when compared to prolonged use of pain medications, which can have serious adverse effects on the liver and kidneys. In PrP, it is the patient's own platelets that are used and Prolotherapy involves the use of only dextrose and a local anesthetic.

The chances of anything going wrong with these treatments are extremely minimal. As we can see, regenerative medicine is the next "Big Thing" in clinical medicine. The next decade will be a decade of the Regenerative Revolution.

CASE STUDY 14

Prabhu was a 45-year-old bank employee who was suffering from long-standing pain in the left foot. He was a diabetic for the last 7 years on oral medication. He was also leading a sedentary lifestyle, and as a result, he was overweight. The pain in the left leg had been there for about three years. After he had been diagnosed to have diabetes, Prabhu had started going for a walk four or five times a week. He noticed that he developed the pain shortly thereafter.

He attributed his pain to the unaccustomed exercise and thought that the pain would soon go away. He applied some pain balm, but the pain was persisting. His son advised him to change his footwear and get some comfortable shoes for walking. On changing his footwear, the pain seemed to get better for a few days, but once again it recurred. He found that the pain always seemed more intense during cold weather. He went to see an orthopedic surgeon who suspected it to be an ankle sprain. He was prescribed some pain killers and was asked to rest and refrain from putting weight on the affected foot. He was also advised to use an elastic crepe bandage to support his ankle for two weeks.

None of these measures helped him. He consulted other specialists who advised that he undergo physiotherapy sessions to control the pain. Prabhu did not experience any relief from his pain. \The pain seemed to be severe in the mornings and then slightly reduced as the day wore on.

On the advice of sundry family members and friends, he applied everything from oils and lotions and massaged his foot, all to no avail. He became extremely wary about going out on social visits as he felt his left ankle was not strong.

He would go to work and then return home. He was quite depressed about the pain. When he came to us at Alleviate, we did a thorough assessment and then diagnosed him to have Achilles tendonitis. He underwent three sessions of PrP therapy and four sessions of Prolotherapy. As is the practice at Alleviate, he was given dietary advice by our nutritionist and put on a weight loss regime. He also attended regular sessions of physical therapy once the PrP plus Prolotherapy sessions were completed. His blood sugar levels stabilized. They had been fluctuating before this. He lost some weight but still had not reached his goal weight. After four to five months, he was able to experience considerable relief from the pain. The ankle strength was also much improved and he was able to walk without difficulty.

As can be seen in Prabhu's case, Prolotherapy helped in reducing and reversing the pain of Achilles tendonitis to a large extent. The multidisciplinary approach of weight loss and physiotherapy also went toward consolidating the healing benefits of PrP Prolotherapy.

In Achilles tendonitis, the Prolotherapy injection is given around the degenerate Achilles tendon to promote tissue regeneration and healing. PrP injections help in the healing process by using concentrated growth factors.

CASE STUDY 15

Sunil was a 23-year-old sportsperson. He was a skater, and he had developed a pain in his right knee a few months ago. It was a dull aching pain that was mainly felt when he climbed upstairs or when he sat down or stood up.

At times the right knee appeared to be a bit swollen as well, but this was not always discernible. He went for an orthopedic consultation and after undergoing all the assessments, he was told that he probably had a muscle pull. He was prescribed some pain medication and was told to rest his knee and apply an ice pack intermittently. The pain was not too severe, but it was a nagging pain. He was unable to give his best efforts to his sport and this was worrying him. As he said, "I know there is nothing seriously wrong with me, but the persistent pain is worrisome." When he came to Alleviate through the recommendation of his physical trainer, we were able to diagnose his condition as Runner's knee or Iliotibial Band Syndrome. He was advised to undergo three sessions of PrP plus Prolotherapy, which he did. The pain completely disappeared following this therapy. In fact, after the treatment, he even represented the country in his event and won a bronze medal. Regenerative medicine offers a nonoperative solution for persistent pain caused by Iliotibial Band Syndrome. Let us learn a little more about this condition.

Iliotibial Band (ITB) Syndrome

ITB Syndrome is a term that is used to refer to any of the several conditions that affect the patella or the kneecap. Any activity that causes repeated stress to the knee joint can result in ITB Syndrome. Some of these activities are running, walking, biking, skating, and cycling. ITB Syndrome is seen more commonly in women, especially if they are overweight.

Symptoms: Pain can occur in the knee on performing activities like walking, climbing up or descending stairs, squatting, kneeling, running, or sitting for a prolonged period with the knee bent.

In the case of ITB syndrome, the pain will be more intense on the outer aspect of the knee joint. It can be caused by overuse of the joint. It can also occur when the thigh muscles are too weak or too tight. Trauma to the knee cap can also lead to the development of ITB Syndrome.

Diagnosis: The condition is mainly diagnosed based on a thorough history and physical examination. Imaging techniques such as X-ray, MRI, and CT scans can aid in the diagnosis of the condition.

Treatment: Conservative Management: The initial step in treating Runner's Knee is the RICE treatment. This includes the following as we already saw in the previous chapter: Rest, Ice, Compression, and Elevation. Pain medication such as Ibuprofen can help reduce pain and inflammation. Apart from this, based on the underlying condition, the treatment will be tailored by the doctor for each patient.

The patient may be advised some strengthening exercises and shoe inserts if required. For ITB syndrome, specifically, as well the same conservative measures are recommended. Surgical Management: In persistent cases of ITB syndrome, where there is tightening of the band, surgical release is recommended as a last resort.

Regenerative therapy: This is a non-surgical alternative for the management of ITB syndrome. PrP plus Prolotherapy stimulates the body to repair all the supportive ligaments attached to the knee joint. It plays a role in healing the iliotibial band and promoting cartilage regeneration. It is generally considered a safe therapy for the management of ITB syndrome.

Lax Ligaments and Joints

Ligaments are bands of connective tissue that connect bones and provide stability to the joints. They are usually tight enough to provide support to the bones and joints.

At times they may be lax. This condition is also referred to as loose joints or joint laxity. Ligament laxity can affect any joint in the body, such as those in the neck, shoulders, ankles, or knees.

Symptoms: A lax ligament can result in frequent injuries or dislocations of the joint. There may be an increased range of movement at the affected joint known as hypermobility. The person may experience pain, numbness, or tingling in and around the joint. Muscle spasms may be seen around the joints as well.

There are some medical conditions that affect the connective tissues in the body and cause generalized joint laxity. Apart from that, joint laxity is commonly seen in athletes who perform specific sports like gymnastics. Lax ligaments if left untreated for long can give rise to early arthritis and the degenerative cascade.

Treatment: Prolotherapy is the treatment of choice to tighten lax or loose ligaments. When prolotherapy is administered to the fibro-osseous junctions, it causes inflammation. This stimulates the fibroblasts to synthesize new collagen fibers, thereby tightening the lax ligaments. As we have seen, Regenerative Therapies can help alleviate chronic pain to a very large extent. They can bring about healing and restoration without the need for drastic surgical measures. They have a huge role to play in the coming years to ensure everyone is able to lead a pain-free active lifestyle.

At Alleviate we provide these recent advances in chronic pain management. If you or your loved one is suffering from chronic pain and you do not know where to go, having been to all the specialists, I would urge you to visit us. We would assess the patient completely and suggest therapies tailor-made for them. We also follow the multidisciplinary approach at Alleviate. This ensures that along with pain therapy, the general health of the patient is taken care of too.

Precepts and Precautions

1. The next decade will most likely witness the regenerative revolution.

153

2. Instead of specialist hopping, those suffering from chronic pain will consult pain specialists.
3. Regenerative therapy triggers the natural healing capacity of the body.
4. PrP plus Prolotherapy: Effective in reducing chronic pain with almost no side effects.
5. Management of chronic pain should include a multidisciplinary approach: dietary advice, physiotherapy, clinical counseling, etc.
6. Neglecting any disease or pain can eventually lead to bigger issues.

9

TO OPERATE OR NOT/SURGERY—YES OR NO?

A stitch in time saves nine

The idea of undergoing surgical therapy for any illness brings about different reactions in different people. There are many who will want to avoid having surgery due to their reluctance for going under the knife. Then there are those who may consider surgical management and the advances in this field to be a godsend and a boon. They would probably argue that surgical treatments are the best option and surgery can negate the need for time-consuming conservative therapy and can bring about the reversal of the disease condition in one stroke. Of course, there is no doubt that surgical management of illnesses is definitely a boon. Numerous life-threatening conditions can be managed by this method of treatment and the quality of life of people can be improved in many others. So, is a stitch in time always the better choice?

The keyword here is 'IN TIME.' While surgery, no doubt, has an important role to play in modern medicine, it is also equally important to take into account a few other factors such as indications, prognosis, stage of disease, and the present level of

155

disability. These aspects are all the more important when we talk of surgery for degenerative joint disorders.

Chettinad is an area in Tamil Nadu where you have more than 70 villages, each having numerous century-old houses, the traditional Chettinad residences. If you walk through the streets of any of these villages, you will see some of these houses resplendent with their shiny colorful paint and polished wooden doors. At the same time, there are many houses that look quite rundown with their faded paintwork, cracked tiles, and damaged woodwork.

Let us visit the homes of two people Mr. Ramesh Palaniappan and Mr. Shiva Alagappan.

Ramesh's house is situated in the village of Devakottai. It is a sprawling traditional Chettinad residence. The home is used by various members of the family for conducting all their family functions, ceremonies, weddings, receptions, etc. As the house has people living there, it is maintained very well. The huge mansion is cleaned regularly. In keeping with the Chettinad tradition, Ramesh's home, too, has a lot of superior quality glass, tiles, and marble. There is a lot of woodwork and brassware as well. Although the wood used is Burma teak, if it is not maintained properly it can lead to termite infestation. Ramesh takes great pride in his home and ensures that each maintenance task is carried out at the right time. The walls are painted or whitewashed at regular intervals.

The extensive woodwork is inspected regularly and dusted and polished as required. The brassware is kept shiny with weekly polishing. Damaged roof tiles are promptly replaced and any leakage or water seepage is promptly attended to as well.

All appliances are kept in working order and the plumbing is checked regularly. Because of the meticulous periodic care lavished on the house, the house has aged well, and is a pleasure to live in and visit. It has not needed any major renovation work.

Shiva's ancestral home, too, is in the same village, two lanes away. Until recently, there was nobody in residence, and the house was locked up most of the time. During his parent's time, the house was used now and then for a family vacation or a religious ceremony, but as the years passed, the visits of the family decreased. With many of them now living either abroad or in other states, the house hardly had any visitors. The caretaker entrusted with looking after the house too ceased staying there on a permanent basis, and of late, visited the house once in a while just to ensure there were no encroachments or trespassers.

When Shiva visited the place after a gap of many years, he was shocked to see how rundown it had become. With the help of his childhood friend Ramesh, he set about restoring the home to its former glory. He was able to get the services of all the expert workmen and artisans who regularly worked on the maintenance of Ramesh's home. The interior of the house was as bad as the exterior. The whole interior was filled with dust and cobwebs. The roof tiles were broken in many places leading to water seepage. This had caused fungus growth on the walls. Some of the woodwork and pillars were infested with termites. The plumbing had eroded and had to be changed entirely with fresh piping. The walls had to be scrapped and redone extensively and repainted. The woodwork too required termite treatment from those experienced in pest control. Some of the precious antique furniture was unsalvageable and had to be discarded. Restoring the house to its former glory cost Shiva quite a bit. Negligence can end up costing one a pretty penny, be it a house or your body.

When problems are attended to then and there, drastic measures can be avoided to a large extent. This is especially true when we look at the lifecycle or the progression of a degenerative disease condition in the joints.

Degenerative joint disease is usually initiated while the patient is in their 30s or 40s. It usually starts with mild symptoms and the severity of the disease increases slowly. Degenerative conditions are known for their long period of progression. There is also a gradual increase both in the frequency and in the intensity of pain associated with the degenerative condition.

Eventually, it leads to a restriction in the daily activities of life for the affected person. If unchecked or untreated at this stage, the disease can go on to cause disability or deformity. The quality of life of the patient can get compromised. This is the sequence of events that a degenerative condition can go through if not treated on time.

The question here is this: when and how can surgery help in this situation?

As we saw in the analogy of the two houses, drastic measures are indicated when there is neglect. The same applies in the case of degenerative joint conditions as well. Early treatment with the various modalities available can definitely prevent or delay the need for surgical management.

In our country, negligence of a degenerative disease condition is mainly due to the callous attitude toward the disease. As it is perceived as a non-life-threatening condition, not much attention is given to its management. The treatment at best is haphazard with remedies being adopted for immediate pain relief.

Also in our Indian society, unsound advice from friends, relatives, and neighbors plays a huge role in the faulty management of these disease conditions. Every well-meaning acquaintance has a solution that he/she swears by. Our poor patient faithfully tries one after another in the proverbial hunt for the golden pot at the end of the rainbow. In the meantime, the degenerative process runs its course unhampered.

However, I must emphasize the following points:

1. Every case of arthritis does not mandate total knee/hip replacement.
2. Every case of sciatica does not mandate disc surgery.

3.   Every person in chronic pain does not require surgery for getting better.

Having said that, one should also be aware that there are certain situations or indications where a patient will definitely benefit from surgical therapy. The trick is to identify the right indications and the right timing for surgical management. Surgery performed at the RIGHT TIME and for the RIGHT REASONS will give the maximum benefit to a patient suffering from degenerative joint disease. Surgery performed for proper reasons with correct indications can be a life-changing event for patients suffering from chronic degenerative disease of the joints. It can improve their quality of life and change it for the better. The following two case studies will help highlight the importance of the indications for surgery and the timing of surgery in degenerative joint disorders.

CASE STUDY 16

Deepan and Manoj are two patients, both in their 30s, who were suffering from low back pain, with radiating pain to the legs. On being investigated, they both were found to have lower lumbar intervertebral disc herniation leading to sciatica pain. Both of them were found to be overweight and in poor physical health. They were also following a sedentary lifestyle. After the diagnosis, Deepan was willing to make drastic changes in his lifestyle. He was treated with transforaminal epidural injections for the back pain.

He immediately began following a weight loss diet and regular exercising and was able to decrease his weight considerably in six months. However, it took two years of regular diet and exercise to reach his goal weight, that is, his ideal body weight. He also underwent regular physiotherapy and diligently followed spine-strengthening exercises.

As a result of his concerted and consistent efforts, he was soon able to return to an active life. Fast forward to the present, 15 years later, he has absolutely no problems with his back. He has maintained his weight and his physical condition by keeping to the lifestyle changes he made. Apart from that single episode of back pain, he has not experienced any pain involving his spine. There was no indication at any time for him to undergo any surgical procedure for his back pain.

Manoj, on the other hand, was totally averse to turning his life around by adopting a healthier lifestyle. He was much too focused on his career and was unwilling to put in the required amount of consistent effort that Deepan had put in. Moreover, he had been wrongly advised by some well-meaning relatives that disc problems were never resolved with conservative management, and surgical approach was the best way to deal with disc prolapse. He, therefore, opted to undergo discectomy and lumbar fusion surgery. He said he was looking for a quick permanent fix for his back pain.

However, he did not give any importance to post-surgery rehabilitation, weight loss, or regular physical exercise. He expected the back surgery to have provided the 'magic cure' and did not deem it necessary to take any effort on his part. Taking for granted that all was well with his spine, he even resorted to lifting heavy furniture at home on occasion.

This lackadaisical attitude resulted in him developing failed back surgery syndrome in four years. In simple terms, we can describe this as a situation where the spine surgery did not yield the result that the patient expected. Manoj continued to experience low back pain, which severely impacted his quality of life. When we see the treatment undertaken by Deepan and Manoj, it is easy to figure out that Deepan followed the right line of treatment. In Manoj's case, surgery on the spine was not warranted at that time. He was young, and his condition could have been managed excellently with conservative methods. A little effort on his part to change his existing lifestyle along with regular exercise would have brought about good results.

In this situation, the timing of the surgery was not correct. Surgery should have been used as a later option, only if other conservative treatments failed to relieve his back pain.

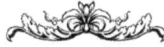

CASE STUDY 17

Here, I want to present two patients, Mr. Gopinath, 64 years old, and Mr. Shekhar, 67 years old. They are both active people, in fairly good health, with minor comorbidities. However, in the recent period, both have been diagnosed to have stage 4 arthritis of the hip joints. Given their age, lack of any serious comorbidities, stage of arthritis, severity of pain, and restricted mobility, and the severe restrictions imposed on the quality of life by the disease, both of them could be considered ideal candidates for undergoing total hip replacement (THR) surgery.

However, only Gopinath opted to undergo THR. He also followed up with proper supervised postsurgical rehabilitative measures. He was given regular physiotherapy and he underwent several sessions of hydrotherapy as well.

He was diligent in carrying out the hip muscle strengthening exercises advised by the physiotherapist. It has been 5 years since he underwent THR and he has had a fairly uneventful recovery period. He is pain-free and is able to move on his own with ease. His quality of life has definitely improved for the better.

Shekhar, on the other hand, decided to not go for THR. He was frightened off of the surgery after listening to some friends who gave their half-baked advice with a lot of exaggeration.

This made him reluctant to go under the knife, although THR would have benefitted him greatly. He managed to pull on with pain killers for a while, even as the pain worsened and his mobility kept deteriorating. He needed help for most of his activities of daily living.

In a couple of years, he began to compensate for the affected joint by putting extra weight on the other side. This in turn led to worsening of arthritis in the other hip and knee joint as well. Eventually, he developed sacroiliac joint pain and was restricted to a wheelchair. In five years, his condition had worsened considerably. Had Shekhar opted to undergo THR on the affected side, the damage to the hip and knee joints on the other side could have been prevented. Timely surgery saved Gopinath from putting an increased load on the other hip and knee joint, and also prevented him from developing sacroiliac joint pain.

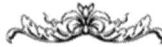

From the above two case studies, it is clear that surgery definitely has a role to play in chronic pain associated with degenerative conditions of the joint. The two main questions to be kept in mind while making a decision are as follows:

(a) Is surgery warranted for the condition?
(b) Is it the right time for the surgery?

When a disease has progressed extensively and is not amenable to any of the other nonsurgical methods in reducing pain, then surgical management is definitely indicated. The benefits of surgery should exceed or outweigh any negative impact or after-effects of the surgical procedure. The benefits of surgery should far exceed the results seen with other modes of therapy.

The surgery should hold the promise of restoring mobility or function to the extent not achieved with other conservative means of treatment. We must be reasonably sure that the patient's quality of life would improve post-surgery to the extent not possible with conservative management.

Coming back to our analogy, we can say without a doubt that regular maintenance of a house can ensure structural strength and render the place livable at all times. The same holds true for our bodies as well. The right treatment taken at the right time holds the key to recovering our health. For this, we need a correct diagnosis of our condition as well as a proper assessment of the level of morbidity. Only then can an accurate decision regarding surgery be taken. At Alleviate, our highly trained professional team of Orthopedic Surgeons, Physiotherapists, Lifestyle consultants, etc., can help assess and guide you in the proper treatment approach.

Precepts and Precautions

1. Ensure that your disease condition warrants a surgical procedure.
2. Is the pain worsening every year? Is the pain unbearable?
3. Ensure that you do not have other serious comorbidities that can make surgery a risk.
4. Is your disease seriously hampering your quality of life? Is the disease limiting your mobility?
5. Learn about how much improvement you can expect from the surgical procedure.
6. Make sure you are committed to following all the postsurgical rehabilitation therapies as advised by your doctor or physiotherapist.

10

EXERCISE AND PHYSICAL THERAPY: ONE DAY AT A TIME

An invaluable investment toward your future

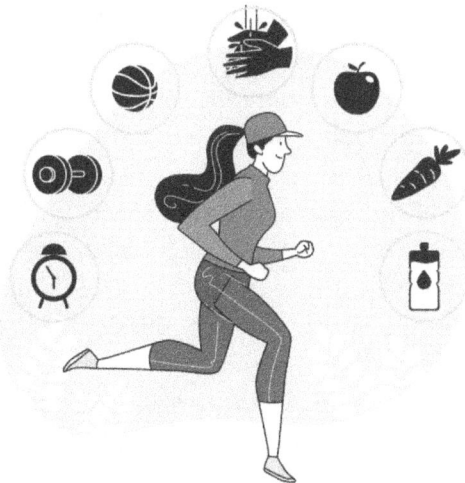

The terms exercise and physical activity are familiar to everyone. You would have come across numerous articles in books and magazines extolling the benefits of regular exercise. Or your doctor might have advised you about the same.

We listen to the advice, make up our minds to follow that advice, and maybe even actually do it for some time. But most of us soon lose that initial momentum and enthusiasm. This could happen for various reasons. Maybe, being over-enthusiastic, you chose an exercise regime or physical activity that is simply not possible to keep at. For instance, you might have decided you would go for a 10 KM walk every day; that is a very difficult goal to reach daily if you are a person who has a busy work schedule or a busy professional career. Another reason for giving up on exercising would be not seeing immediate results. If you started walking in the mornings daily with the goal of losing weight, you are not going to see tangible results within a few days or a couple of weeks.

So before setting our exercise or physical activity goals, we should be clear in our minds about the timeframe in which we want this to happen. Setting unrealistic timeframes will lead to disinterest and cessation of the activity.

We must learn to look at exercise and physical therapy as an investment. It is like investing small amounts of money regularly, which grows to a tidy amount over a period of time. People, in general, give a lot of importance to wealth creation during their lifetime. They look closely into the ways and means by which they can increase their wealth. They invest their time and energy in pursuing a career that serves to not only meet their immediate needs but also would help them reach their financial goals. They put a lot of thought and effort into investing their money wisely. This is termed compounding your wealth. So, even if they would have started out with a small amount of wealth or money, the continuous regular additions to their investments result in a large amount. This is what we term compounding wealth. It is considered a very powerful principle of wealth creation.

You can end up with an amount substantially greater than what you started out with as a result of sustained effort, dedication, increased awareness and knowledge about the field, and wisdom and experience gained through the years. Similarly, we must make regular efforts toward compounding our health.

There are various methods or paths that we can follow to lead a healthy life. Physical activity and regular exercise are two of the important ways in which you can ensure you remain healthy. By exercising regularly and following some pattern of physical activity, we are making regular investments toward our health. I call this compounding our health.

"Those who think they have not time for bodily exercise, will sooner or later have to find time for illness." These words attributed to a British aristocrat from the 19th century, Lord Edward Stanley, ring true even to this day. Regular physical activity can be said to be a 'wonder drug.' It helps not only in maintaining good health but also in the recovery from many illnesses. One situation where exercise plays a huge role is after childbirth. Regular exercise after delivery can help in promoting weight loss and boosting the energy levels of the new mother. It helps to strengthen the lax and stretched abdominal muscles following pregnancy. Physical activity can even reduce stress and symptoms of postpartum.

CASE STUDY 17

Viji and Reema are both second-time mothers in their early thirties. Let us take a look at their post-delivery journeys. Viji was 32 years old when she delivered her second baby through normal delivery. She had an episiotomy to facilitate the delivery. Episiotomy is an incision made in the perineum to deliver the baby easily and to prevent other harmful tears or damage. This incision is then sutured after the baby is born. The episiotomy wound heals in about a week or 10 days. Viji did not have any family members to help out after her delivery and she was forced to return to her normal household chores within a week after having her baby.

She was immersed in looking after her family and totally neglected her health. Looking after the needs of her 6-year-old daughter and her newborn son took up all her time. She did not even go for her post-natal check-up. She told herself that she would recover just fine. As a result of totally neglecting her health, she never got back to her pre-pregnancy weight. Nor did she ever do any pelvic floor muscle strengthening exercises. Eventually, she began experiencing back pain. This too, she did not take seriously, and attributed it to normal post-pregnancy effects. She assumed she would soon be back to her normal self.

The slow deterioration in her health due to lack of self-care and proper physical exercise began. And now, around 15 years down the line, she is suffering from obesity and, more distressing, incontinence. The incontinence was a result of not having done pelvic floor exercises after her delivery. It has affected her quality of life to a great extent. Reema too delivered her second child when she was 34 years old. She had a normal delivery with an episiotomy, but the difference was she took her health very seriously. She was very careful to wait until the episiotomy wound had healed before exerting herself. She was very conscious about going for her postnatal check-up.

Once she got her gynecologist's thumbs-up, she started her exercise schedule. Initially, she started a Kegel exercise regime. These exercises help to strengthen the pelvic floor muscles and prevent the development of incontinence. Along with that, she ensured that she was involved in some sort of regimented physical activity always. She went for Pilates and Aerobics sessions in turn. She was always including some cardiovascular or muscle strengthening and toning activity in her daily schedule. And now, years later, she is enjoying a very good quality of life. She is able to give her best to her family and to her profession. Looking after her health and physical fitness has paid off with rich dividends in her case.

From the above two scenarios, one can understand how much difference regular exercise and physical therapy can make to a person's quality of life. The stark difference between the two women with regard to their quality of life clearly stands out. While Reema is out enjoying her annual holidays with her husband and children, Viji is hesitant to even leave her home for short periods fearing an embarrassing situation due to the incontinence.

Role Of Physiotherapy In Patient Recovery

Regular exercise and physical therapy have a huge role to play in recovery from ailments as well. This holds especially true when it comes to recovery from musculoskeletal or joint problems. Physiotherapy helps the patient to recover movement and function of the affected muscle or joint following an injury or a treatment procedure like surgery or splinting in a case of fracture. Physiotherapists assess a patient who comes following surgery or some other treatment or those who come after an illness. They identify the particular issues that need to be addressed and provide tailor-made therapy regimes for the patient. They work closely with the treating physician or surgeon to ensure that the therapy plan is suitable and in no way detrimental or contraindicated for the patient.

Physiotherapists play a huge role in the continuum of care for the patient and also support the family members by teaching them home exercises that they can encourage the patient to follow. Especially, in situations where the patient has a chronic ailment or his/her mobility is severely restricted, the physiotherapist is the main encourager and motivator to keep up the daily exercises and stretching routines. Musculoskeletal physiotherapy helps in pain management. The physiotherapist helps in addressing not only pain, but also other symptoms, such as muscle weakness, loss of stability, and loss of function and ability.[5]

---

[5]https://www.longdom.org/open-access/physiotherapy-for-musculoskeletal-problems-in-primary-health-care-87431.html

Trained physiotherapists help the patients to develop coping techniques to deal with the pain and also with the loss of function or mobility that they are experiencing. They also formulate completely custom-made and feasible maintenance physical therapy exercise schedules that the patient can follow easily. They help the patient to set short-term goals that they can reach, which act as additional encouragement to continue with the therapy. In short, sustained and dedicated physical therapy can speed up the healing process considerably in a patient and make A return to routine activities.

CASE STUDY 19

This is a case study of two men, both in their early thirties, who underwent treatment for a knee injury.

Dilip and Kishen are both in their thirties. They came to us at Alleviate at different times, albeit with very similar problems. Both of them had suffered partial thickness tears of the anterior cruciate ligaments and severe strain along with meniscus injury and collateral ligament damage as well.

Both of them were treated with comprehensive PrP and Prolotherapy sessions. They were advised multiple sessions, which they completed. Further, they were advised to undergo physical therapy for strengthening of the quadriceps and hamstring muscles. Quadriceps is a large muscle group comprising four muscles that cover the front of the thigh and help in standing, walking, running, etc. They also help to stabilize the knee cap. The hamstrings, on the other hand, are a group of three muscles present posteriorly in the thigh. These muscles help mainly in bending the knee. They are also involved in some movements of the hip joints as well.

As mentioned, both Dilip and Kishen underwent the PrP plus Prolotherapy sessions. However, following these sessions, Dilip did not continue to attend the physiotherapy sessions. He did not take the requirement for exercise and rehabilitation seriously. Anterior cruciate ligament injuries are known to be usually accompanied by some quadriceps wasting as well. Not doing the muscle strengthening exercises led to further weakening of his quadriceps muscle.

This led to ligament instability in the knee joint on the affected side. All these factors of pain, lack of exercise and physical therapy, lack of movement, weakening of the quadriceps muscle, and instability of ligaments led to his developing knee joint instability on the affected side and degenerative changes in the joints. He eventually ended up developing arthritic changes in the knee joint while in his late thirties.

Kishen, however, took his health seriously. He made an effort to understand the working mechanism of the knee joint and was keen to get started on the treatment regime. He was mentally committed to doing his part to the best of his ability. Once the PrP Prolotherapy sessions were completed, he was diligent in continuing the physical therapy sessions.

The regular effort on his part to perform the muscle strengthening exercises and attend the physical therapy sessions paid off. In just a year's time, the injured knee was much stronger than the other knee. In my practice, I have seen quite a few patients like Kishen. This only happens when the patient is dedicated and disciplined toward strengthening the affected muscles and toward exercise and physical therapy. An injury can actually, under these circumstances, lead to such a positive result, where arthritis in the affected knee gets better and the knee is in a better shape compared to the normal one. As mentioned before, at Alleviate, we follow the multidisciplinary approach. This means, whatever interventions are carried out by the pain physicians or orthopedic surgeons, they are combined with patient education on the importance of rehabilitation, which involves physical therapy and exercise.

The patients are encouraged to initially attend the physical therapy sessions in the clinic under the supervision and guidance of our trained physical therapists. This helps them learn the exercise routine so that they can practice the same at home correctly. If necessary, the relatives are taught these exercises as well, so that they can help the patients at home.

Role Of Exercise In Managing Chronic Pain

You may wonder, how exactly does exercise help when one is in pain? Will exercise not exacerbate an already painful condition? You would be partially right. Exercise can be painful when a person is already suffering from a painful condition like fibromyalgia. However, exercise and physical activity, when used within the specified parameters of frequency, duration, and intensity have been said to significantly improve chronic pain. This means the prescribed exercise should be performed only as often as the physical therapist recommends. The length of time and the physical effort by the patient must be regulated as well. Exercise has been offered as one of the rehabilitation measures for patients suffering from chronic pain due to conditions such as fibromyalgia, myofascial pain, and many other chronic musculoskeletal conditions as we have seen through all the earlier chapters.

Research has also established that exercise is indeed beneficial in chronic painful conditions. In fact, physical inactivity can add to the debility in patients suffering from chronic pain. Exercise is said to reduce pain perception. Research has shown that when one is suffering from a chronic painful condition if you undertake a single session of physical activity, it is bound to exacerbate the pain. However, regular exercise has the benefit of reducing pain perception. In chronic painful conditions, exercise not only has a beneficial effect on pain, but also helps to improve sleep, physical functioning, and coping with the disease condition. Poor sleep can actually exacerbate the symptoms of pain, fatigue, and stiffness in chronic pain patients.

Structured physical activity helps these patients experience a higher quality of sleep. In fact, one study has reported that exercise was found to relieve pain and improve physical function and quality of life. It reduces the risk of developing comorbidities, such as hypertension, obesity, and osteoporosis. Frequent movement is definitely better than sedentary behavior.

Role Of Regular Exercise In Health

Due to all the awareness created on social media, these days all of us know and agree that regular exercise is beneficial to us. However, knowing and actually practicing the same are two very different things. It has been said that physical fitness not only contributes to a healthy body but also helps us be mentally fit and increases our creativity. Regular physical activity is said to have immediate as well as long-term health benefits. Regular physical activity can definitely improve one's quality of life.

When you start an exercise routine today, it is something your future self will thank you for. Exercising reduces the risk of developing many of the chronic illnesses seen in our society in the present age, such as diabetes, hypertension, and obesity. It can in fact be termed as a miracle cure that is not only easily accessible and free but also has proven to be effective. A lot of people say that beginning their day with physical activity of some kind helps them to maintain a happy and positive frame of mind throughout the day. It is also equally important to be aware of the other side of the coin.

Inactivity or a sedentary lifestyle has been proved to be dangerous. Some have termed inactivity as a silent killer. It can actually increase the risk of developing a life-threatening illness such as stroke or heart attack. It can lead to obesity as well. Even if you are doing some sort of physical activity every day, if you spend the rest of the day lying down, that can still be bad for your health. So, how can you make physical activity a part of your daily life? Of course, taking part in sports and games or joining a regimented exercise schedule at a gym can be very effective.

However, that is not the only way. You can start with small but daily steps. For one, you can start walking every day. Avoid using your car to travel short distances and walk or cycle instead.

The physical activity that you indulge in should increase your heart rate and your respiratory rate. Basically, that means your heart beats faster and you breathe faster as well. A physical activity that can be termed moderate-intensity or high-intensity will only be beneficial to your health. A casual slow stroll through the park may not be as effective. An exercise of moderate intensity will allow you to talk, but you probably cannot sing while performing it. However, when you are performing a vigorous or high-intensity workout, you will not be able to speak even a few words before pausing to catch your breath. Of course, a vigorous activity will definitely bring more benefit than that offered by moderate activity. But not everyone can undertake to do these kinds of physical activities.

Benefits of regular exercise:

1. Prevents excessive weight gain
2. Helps maintain weight loss
3. Prevents/reduces high blood pressure
4. Improves muscle strength
5. Improves physical stamina
6. Helps control the blood sugar levels
7. Reduces bad cholesterol levels in the blood
8. Promotes blood circulation
9. Reduces risk of many cancers
10. Elevates your mood
11. Boosts one's confidence and improves self-esteem
12. Improves memory and recall
13. Improves the quality of sleep and relaxation
14. Reduces chronic pain and improves pain tolerance

The list is endless actually! Phew! Why would someone not want to start exercising on a regular basis?

If you want to be healthy and live life to the fullest, you should start exercising as well. It can be anything from a 30-minute brisk walk to a supervised session at the local gym. There are numerous kinds of exercises that one can follow to keep it from being monotonous or boring: Pilates, Aerobics, Zumba. Choose the one that appeals to you. You can even alternate between different routines, but it is important you start one.

If you are recovering from an illness or you are above the age of 45, you should consult your doctor to find out what kind of exercises are suitable for you. If you plan to start an exercise schedule for the first time, it is better to have some sort of pre-exercise screening. This can help detect any cardiac or respiratory issues that need to be taken care of. If so, the doctor might recommend the level of activity that you can safely perform. Pregnant women should take the advice of their gynecologist before starting any exercise routines. However, in a normal pregnancy, simple walking is encouraged.

Even after deciding to start on a daily physical activity or exercise routine, some people have difficulty in following the same. The initial enthusiasm soon wears off.

And then, one might not really feel up to performing at the same level every day. Below are some tips you can follow that will help you keep your resolve.

1. The beginning is the hardest part. Once you start, it gets easier. You need the motivation to get started, but the habit will keep you going.
2. Set realistic goals. It is best to start with easy-to-achieve goals and when you are sure you can reach them, then set bigger goals.
3. Set weekly goals instead of daily goals. This way you can always make up for a bad day and you will not feel demotivated.
4. There are a number of devices that can help track your activity. For example, smartwatches can track your footsteps. This is a good way of keeping count.

5. Being part of a group can be motivating. Join a group of friends as you exercise; you will not even notice the effort when you are with others.

6. In spite of your best efforts, you might fail and miss your target due to many reasons. Do not let that discourage you. Someone once said, "Failure is only when you fail to get up after falling." Start anew and keep going.

The key point here is you must fix an exercise or physical activity routine that is feasible and possible for you. When you start with small and consistent steps, success is sure to follow. Remember, any exercise is better than no exercise.

Therefore, if on certain days you cannot undertake moderate-intensity or high-intensity activities, go for a simple stroll before you end the day. It will be a stress reliever. Exercise or physical activity is said to release endorphins that can make you feel relaxed and happy.

11

ROLE OF NUTRITION IN CHRONIC PAIN

"Let food be thy medicine"

– Hippocrates!

We have all heard the common adage, 'You are what you eat." The French lawyer Anthelme Brillat-Savarin once said, *"Tell me what you eat and I will tell you what you are."* The role of nutrition in maintaining good health has been extensively studied. The importance of making healthy food choices is clear to most people as it is a widely discussed topic these days. It is indeed true that what we eat affects our health to a great extent. Our body is constantly in a phase of growth, repair, and regeneration. All the cells in our body that make up the various tissues and organs such as the hair, skin, muscle, and bone have a set life span. For example, the skin cells live for about a month and the red blood cells for about four months. Proper nutrition is required for all cellular functions to happen optimally. The health of the new cells that are being made depends on the nutritional status of our body.

When we follow a healthy dietary pattern, the cells being synthesized are healthy also. Imbalance or deficiency in any of the macro- or micronutrients can lead to derangement of the cell functions. Persistent nutrient deficiency can cause permanent illness.

Role Of Nutrition In Healing/Running On Empty

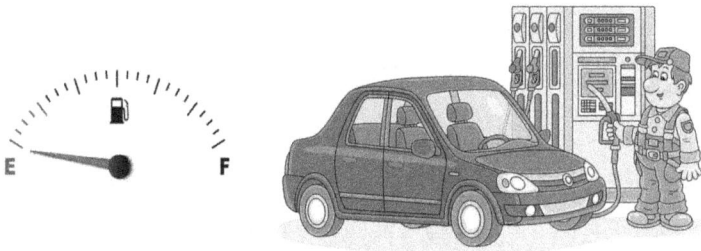

The human body has an amazing ability to heal itself after an injury. There are numerous ways in which we see this happening. For example, the damaged lung cells in a smoker renew themselves after he quits smoking. When there is a fracture, we see the bone cells taking up the repair and regeneration process and growing new bone. Or even following a simple cut, platelets in the blood help in stopping the bleeding, and the connective tissue cells help in wound healing.

However, for all these healing processes to take place the body must be healthy and hold adequate reserves of all the nutrients that play a role. Nutrient reserves in the body can be compared to the fuel in your car. What happens when the fuel indicator is hovering over the 'E' mark? You immediately realize that you need to fill up your tank. You might have maintained your car well with regular servicing and all the systems might be functioning well, but if you run out of fuel, your vehicle is not going to move anywhere.

Again, do you know what can happen if you run your vehicle on low fuel levels? Often people ignore the warning light indicating low fuel levels. They want to somehow manage with the remaining fuel for as long as possible. But this can turn out to be a very costly exercise in the end.

If you wait till your fuel tank is absolutely empty before filling up again, you can cause serious damage to your car's fuel pump. It can get over-stressed and overheated due to the lack of lubrication that the fuel actually provides. Your engine too can get damaged by the sludge that is at the bottom of the fuel tank. When you run low on fuel, the sludge can get sucked up by the fuel pump and carried to the engine. This will cause the fuel filter and the injector to get clogged up. Running on low fuel reserves also carries the risk of running completely empty unexpectedly. You might get stalled in the middle of a busy highway or just when you were going for an important engagement.

Again, when you know the fuel tank is near empty, you will drive in a state of heightened tension, anticipating the worst. This anxiety and stress will disturb your mind, and it could even lead to an accident.

Just by ensuring that you have enough fuel in your tank for your car, you can get peace of mind and the assurance that you will have a trouble-free ride and reach your destination without any problems.

The same is true for our bodies as well. A proper, balanced diet means the required amounts of nutrients are reaching your body. Ensuring proper nutrient reserves leads to a healthy body that has the optimum ability to deal with the various stresses it is subject to.

Often when people start feeling tired and lethargic, they attribute it to the aging process. They fail to realize that improper diet is the reason for their symptoms.

Energy Bank

Let us look at some of the nutrients that play a role in reducing fatigue and improving energy levels.

Vitamin D, Vitamin C, magnesium, iron, potassium, Vitamin B12, and the other B-complex vitamins, and zinc are the key micronutrients that are essential for optimal energy in our body. A

healthy nutrient-rich diet can aid in maintaining the natural balance
of our body.

In general, our diet is made of macronutrients and
micronutrients. Foods that we take in large amounts are called
macronutrients. This includes carbohydrates, proteins, and fat.
These food categories form the staple of our diets. They are
responsible for providing energy for our various activities as well as
for the body to build and repair itself. Micronutrients are usually
required by the body in smaller amounts but they are very vital for
the proper functioning of the body. Vitamins, minerals, and trace
elements constitute the micronutrients required by our bodies. They
play an important role in various body functions such as energy
production, blood clotting, and immune function. Minerals play a
vital role in bone health.

In the previous chapters, we have seen the various causes of
chronic pain in the body and the different ways to manage chronic
pain.

Let us now look at how nutritional status impacts chronic pain.

Impact of Diet on Chronic Pain

Chronic pain mainly occurs in the body due to conditions causing
inflammation, stress, or degeneration. In fact, they are inter-related
and may be seen simultaneously in a person having chronic pain

(A) Inflammation: Inflammation is necessary for the body to
fight illness. It is an important part of healing. But
sometimes when the immune function does not work
properly people can be in a constant or recurrent low state
of inflammation. This kind of chronic inflammation is seen
in conditions like rheumatoid arthritis and psoriasis.

(B) Stress: Physical stress in various parts of the body like strains
and sprains can cause chronic pain. Now, these conditions
are exacerbated when a person is overweight or obese.

Maintaining an ideal body weight or BMI is an essential factor for managing chronic pain. Research has shown that people suffering from chronic back pain have high cortisol levels. Foods that decrease cortisol levels can help in controlling chronic low back pain.

Mental stress can also lead to an increased perception of pain. People with mental stress do not eat properly or exercise adequately. This can compound the problem of increased weight and contribute to chronic pain.

(C) Degeneration: Various degenerative changes that occur in the body over time can be a cause of chronic pain. For example, in osteoarthritis of the knee joint, the degenerative changes cause increasing joint pain and stiffness.

It is interesting that nutrition and diet have an impact on all these conditions.

1.   Foods that help reduce inflammation

Food can be either pro-inflammatory or anti-inflammatory. Foods that are pro-inflammatory or that lead to an inflammatory state should be avoided. These include refined carbohydrates, bottled drinks, fried foods, and processed meat. One must avoid eating too much white bread and other bakery products, French fries, burgers with meat patties, sausages, and other processed food. These can be called junk food and it is best to avoid them completely or eat only very occasionally.

Anti-inflammatory foods help bring down the inflammatory state in the body and thereby aid in controlling chronic pain. These include green leafy vegetables, olive oil, nuts, fruits, tomatoes, and fish. Certain fruits and vegetables like apples, blueberries, and leafy greens have high levels of natural antioxidants.

Antioxidants are chemicals that protect the body from free radicals. Free radicals are certain molecules that are formed in our body and they cause damage to the cells. A diet rich in antioxidants can protect the body from many chronic diseases like heart disease and cancer.

2. Maintaining ideal body weight

Ideal body weight seems like an impossible achievement to many. But the benefits of maintaining the correct BMI are many. Having a healthy weight reduces the risk of many chronic illnesses like hypertension, diabetes, and heart disease. When one is overweight or obese, there is increased stress on various organs of the body. The increased stress on the various joints in the body in obese persons leads to chronic pain conditions like arthritis. To maintain an ideal body weight, you must eat a balanced diet. A balanced diet has the right proportion of macronutrients and micronutrients. Your diet must include the right proportion of carbohydrates, proteins, fats, vitamins, minerals, and water. The calorie breakdown for a healthy diet would be carbohydrates 45% to 55%, proteins 20% to 25%, and fat 20% to 25%. However, if you are overweight, then the diet has to be adjusted to include more proteins and fewer carbohydrates. This is best done with the guidance of a trained nutritionist.

Foods that can help in reducing the cortisol levels in our bodies include green tea, probiotics, dark chocolate, avocadoes, and spinach. Decreasing cortisol levels can help in managing chronic pain. A balanced diet helps you face the day and its challenges and reduces anxiety.

3. Foods that help in regeneration

There are certain foods that help in the regeneration and repair of the cells and tissues in our body. It is very important to include these foods in your diet. They include blueberries, broccoli, nuts and seeds, ginger, mushrooms, and seafood. Some of these foods especially help in the regeneration of stem cells in the body.

This is important because stem cells have the function of replacing old and damaged cells in our bodies. Because they have a regenerating function, it is vital that the stem cells in our body are healthy. In osteoarthritis and other conditions where there are degenerative changes in the cartilages, foods that help in cartilage regeneration should be taken. Cartilage has a poor blood supply in the body, and therefore it has a limited self-healing ability. Foods that can help reduce chronic pain in the joints and also aid in cartilage regeneration include omega-3 fatty acids, fish oils, nuts and seeds, colorful fruits, olive oil, lentils and beans, and garlic.

Minerals like Glucosamine and Chondroitin sulfate are said to be helpful in cartilage regeneration, but these should be taken only with your doctor's advice.

Importance of Ideal Body Weight in Managing Chronic Pain

Here, I want to stress that, apart from its role in controlling chronic pain, maintaining an ideal body weight has many benefits: efficient circulation of blood in the body, well-balanced fluid levels, low risk of diabetes, heart disease, and breathing problems, and feeling better about oneself and feeling energetic to make further positive changes.

Let me explain this further by telling you about two of our patients who underwent treatment for chronic knee pain at our clinic, Alleviate.

CASE STUDY 20

Madan came to us at Alleviate with long-standing pain in both his knees. He was 55 years old and worked as a manager in a finance company. He had consulted a number of specialists over the years for his pain. He had been diagnosed to have arthritis in the knee joint and was prescribed some pain killers.

The pain was relieved for a few months as long as he took his pain meds. Eventually, he would discontinue his meds fearing the side effects, and the knee pain would reappear. This cycle went on for a few years. However, he found the pain in his knee joints increasing and it reached the stage where he had difficulty in getting to work and performing his daily activities. When we saw Madan at Alleviate, we performed a thorough examination and all the imaging investigations. He was found to be slightly overweight and borderline hypertensive. On X-ray imaging, there were degenerative changes in both the knee joints, more so in the left knee. We treated him with four to five sessions of PrP plus Prolotherapy. He was also referred to our nutritionist and lifestyle modification expert. He was given counseling about the importance of maintaining an ideal body weight and all its attendant benefits. He was prescribed a proper weight-loss diet. He increased his protein intake and restricted his carbohydrate intake. He was diligent about his daily exercise routine. He also came for regular thrice-a-week physiotherapy sessions at our clinic.

He experienced relief from pain and at the end of six months, there was a remarkable change in his condition. His weight was nearer his goal weight and there was a marked decrease in the knee pain. Previously, he had been able to walk only 500 meters, but now after following the strict exercise protocol, he was walking two to three kilometers every day. His blood pressure too was now normal.

CASE STUDY 21

Ramnath was a 52-year-old businessman, having an import-export business. He had been suffering from severe knee pain for a couple of years. On the advice of his relatives, he had tried traditional remedies like oil massages, but to no avail. He was following a pretty sedentary lifestyle with not much physical activity.

His work too involved just sitting in one place for long periods of time. He resorted to taking over-the-counter pain medications from the pharmacy near his house. He found relief from the pain for a few weeks, but eventually, the pain came back, and it also appeared to be worsening. When he came to us, the pain in his knee joints was severe enough to hamper his walking and his daily activities. On examination, we found that he was overweight and X-ray imaging showed degenerative changes in both knee joints.

We diagnosed his condition as osteoarthritis of both the knee joints. He underwent treatment with PrP plus Prolotherapy. He was given about four to five sessions of the same. He was also given lifestyle modification suggestions. He was advised about weight loss and a diet chart was prepared for him according to his weight loss requirement, by our in-house nutritionist. He initially followed the diet schedule and exercised regularly. He attended a few physiotherapy sessions as well. His pain was moderately reduced and he could walk with some ease. However, Ramnath was not diligent about exercising. He gave up going for walks. He did not attend any further physiotherapy sessions at the clinic.

Moreover, he did not follow the diet chart prepared by the dietician. He gave it up after following it for a few weeks. He was back to his sedentary lifestyle with excessive sitting and eating. When we saw him after six months, his weight had increased by about five kilograms. When he initially came to our clinic, his weight had been 81 kilograms. It was no surprise that the pain in his knee joints had reappeared, and again he was finding it difficult to walk as well as carry out his daily activities.So here we can see two people with the same condition who underwent similar treatment. But there is a drastic difference in the outcomes for both of them after a few months. Why is this so?

In general, we have noted that people who do well after treatment for chronic pain are those who have taken the issues of weight control and proper nutrition seriously. Those who have reduced their body weight to get close to their ideal BMI, have shown better and sustained relief from their painful conditions.

Especially when talking about the knee joints, maintaining the ideal body weight is extremely important for the well-being of the joints. The knee joints bear the weight of the body, and therefore being overweight or obese can cause excessive stress on the bones and the ligaments in the joint, leading to early degenerative changes and chronic pain.

Therefore, to maintain your ideal weight, you need to follow a proper diet with the required nutrients and calories in it.

Role of Diet Counseling

So how can we help you at Alleviate? I have already mentioned in the previous chapters that at Alleviate, we follow a multidisciplinary approach in treating our patients. When a patient comes to us for the management of a chronic painful condition, he undergoes a thorough physical examination, whatever the condition might be. Part of the management includes nutritional assessment and appropriate nutritional and dietary advice from our in-house qualified nutritionist in Alleviate.

Here is what Ms. Pooja Shankar, our in-house clinical nutritionist says: The dietary recommendations are made keeping in mind the patient's age, gender, physical condition, comorbidities if any, and the main condition or disease that brought them to us.

Patients come to Alleviate for treatment of various conditions causing chronic pain and distress. They may have degenerative conditions like osteoarthritis of the hip or knee joints, inflammatory diseases like fibromyalgia, chronic pain following trauma like fractures, chronic pain due to nerve impingement like radiculopathies, etc. Whatever the reason for their visit, they are mainly looking to be relieved from their pain. And one of the points we want them to understand is that a holistic approach to their health is essential for longstanding results. I would like to explain this using three scenarios.

Scenario 1

Let us say we have a patient who comes with early arthritis of the knee joint. He is in his forties and he is within his ideal body weight. He does not have any other comorbidities. In this situation, the patient is not looking for weight loss or gain, but only to maintain a healthy and pain-free lifestyle.

Here, we recommend a normal balanced diet with enough calories depending on his lifestyle. A person following a sedentary lifestyle would require a lower number of daily calories than what a person doing strenuous work would need. So, the diet recommendations would be tailored accordingly. Here, an ideal breakdown of the calorie intake would be 50% to 60% from carbohydrates, 20% to 25% from proteins, and 20% to 25% from fats. We would also advise the patient to take the appropriate quantity of micronutrients, that is, vitamins and minerals, in the diet.

Scenario 2

Now, supposing this same patient was overweight or obese, our dietary recommendations would be focused on helping him lose weight while eating healthy.

For those patients who are above the ideal body weight, the dietary advice would be different. Their focus will be on the numbers on the scale. They would know that a reduction in weight will not only help in managing their chronic pain, but will also make them feel better about themselves. So, the diet recommendations will reflect these requirements. When patients are involved in their treatment for chronic pain, they will also be keen to follow the dietician's advice. These patients are prescribed what is known as a restrictive diet.

We all know that our normal Indian diet is rice-based and this makes it high in carbohydrate content. We advise a low carbohydrate diet for weight loss. We cut down on the calories by decreasing the daily carbohydrate intake. At the same time, the patient should not lose muscle mass.

Therefore, the protein allowance per day is increased. It is kept at 0.9 gm/kg for ideal body weight. Fat intake is also restricted. Fat intake is limited to 20 gm/day. Only unsaturated fats are allowed. The patient is advised not to consume saturated fats or trans-fats. Unsaturated fats are beneficial to us in many ways. They are said to be heart-friendly and can reduce high cholesterol levels. They also have an anti-inflammatory effect.

They can help reduce inflammation in patients with chronic pain. Unsaturated fats can be of two types: monounsaturated fats and polyunsaturated fats. What are the foods that contain both these types of unsaturated fats? Monounsaturated fats can be found in olive oil, peanut oil, nuts such as almonds, seeds such as pumpkin seeds and sesame seeds, etc.

Polyunsaturated fats can be found in sunflower oil, corn oil, walnuts, flax seeds, fish, etc. Fish is rich in Omega-3 fats. We have all heard this term being used extensively these days. So, what are Omega-3 fats? And why is it important in our diet?

Omega-3 fats are polyunsaturated fats that cannot be made in our bodies. They are essential fats, which we need to survive. Therefore, we have to obtain it from an external source. As mentioned earlier, fish is an excellent source of Omega-3 fatty acids. It is also found in nuts and seeds such as walnuts and chia seeds. Omega-3 fats help in reducing inflammation in the body. They also help in preventing the formation of plaques in the arteries. They can raise the 'good' cholesterol in the body and help in reducing blood pressure.

Why do we advise to abstain from consuming trans-fat? What do they do? Trans-fats are formed when vegetable oils are heated in the presence of hydrogen and a catalyst. This is hydrogenated oil. You would have heard this term. Vegetable oils are hydrogenated so that they can stay fresh for a long time and also can be heated repeatedly for use. These oils are mainly used in the fast-food industry and in restaurants for frying, baking, and processing food. Trans-fats are also found in beef and, to a small extent, in dairy products. Trans-fat has been found to increase or create inflammation. That is why it is considered harmful to the body.

Trans-fats also raise the levels of 'bad' cholesterol and decrease the levels of 'good' cholesterol in the body. Consuming trans-fat can increase your chances of developing heart disease, stroke, or diabetes. We also encourage the patients who are looking to lose weight to eat more fruits and add sources of flavonoids to their diet.

Flavonoids are certain plant metabolites that act as antioxidants. Flavonoids are said to provide many benefits to us. They are said to have anti-cancer and anti-inflammatory properties. A diet that includes foods containing flavonoids will, therefore, be helpful to patients suffering from chronic pain. Foods rich in flavonoids include fruits, vegetables, nuts, tea, and wine. These foods are also described as 'superfoods.'

Scenario 3

What if this same patient had some comorbidities like diabetes or hypertension? The diet is structured according to the comorbid disease of the patient. For patients with hypertension, we prescribe a restricted sodium diet. Basically, this means a salt-restricted diet. We advise hypertensive patients to avoid foods with high salt content, such as pickles, papads, and all sorts of preserved or processed foods. Most of the preserved or processed foods are high in salt content. We also advise them to restrict their consumption of green leafy vegetables as the sodium content is high in these as well. Patients with high blood pressure are asked to follow the DASH diet—Dietary Approach to Stop Hypertension. Basically, this includes foods that are low in sodium, increased fruits, restriction of proteins and carbohydrates, and foods rich in antioxidants and phytochemicals.

For a diabetic patient, if is borderline diabetes, I recommend a reversal diet. Here the diabetic state can be reversed and the patient's sugar levels can be normalized. In others, where reversal is not feasible, we give a low carbohydrate diet with low glycemic index (GI) foods, anti-inflammatory foods, and sufficient protein. Basically, low GI foods take longer to raise the patient's blood sugar levels than moderate or high GI foods do. Some of the low GI foods are barley, oats, nonstarchy vegetables, sweet potatoes, and fruits. Chickpeas and raw carrots are also low GI foods.

Diets in Specific Conditions causing Chronic Pain

Let us now see what specific dietary advice we would give for the management of degenerative conditions like arthritis.

The primary aim in these patients is to prevent muscle wasting. When asked to make a 24-hour recall of their diet, it is usually seen that most of these patients are not consuming enough protein in their diet. They are also not getting enough good fats. They follow a sedentary lifestyle with no regular physical activities. There is almost no exposure to sunlight, thereby leading to Vitamin D deficiency. Most of these patients also tend to be overweight.

So along with anti-inflammatory foods, the diet would be aimed at reducing weight with improvement in muscle mass. A decrease in body weight or achieving the ideal BMI can help greatly in pain by reducing the stress on the joints.

Autoimmune disease is another condition where patients suffer from chronic pain. For example, in rheumatoid arthritis patients suffer from pain in the small joints of the hands and feet. The joint lining is affected and this can eventually lead to joint deformity and destruction. For these patients, a diet that includes more unsaturated fats should be provided. The daily dietary recommendation for calorie breakdown would be 60% unsaturated fats, 15% carbohydrates, and 35% proteins. Here the stress would be on high biological value proteins to provide the essential amino acids. High protein intake helps to lower inflammation in these patients.

Systemic lupus erythematosus (SLE) or Lupus as it is commonly called, is another autoimmune disease where there is chronic joint pain, stiffness, and swelling, in addition to a number of other symptoms. Lupus patients benefit greatly from an intermittent fasting diet. This involves an 8-hour window for food intake and a 16-hour fasting period. However, you must follow these diets only after consulting a clinical nutritionist.

Be Hydrated

Water is essential in our body for circulation of the nutrients as well as for the elimination of waste. Keep track of your daily water intake. Ensure that you drink two to three liters of water per day unless it is contraindicated for any reason.

Dehydration can cause increased sensitivity to pain and adequate hydration can aid in healing and pain reduction. Water is indeed the elixir of life.

Along with water intake, ensure that your diet has an adequate amount of fiber as well. This helps in maintaining ideal body weight and in proper digestion of food. Stay away from ultra-processed food and junk food. Also, lower your sugar intake; do not consume bottled sugary drinks. These foods are prone to increase oxidation and inflammation in the body, and thereby increase pain. As you can see, the right nutrition is very critical not only for a healthy life but also in the management of various conditions that present with chronic pain. For this, you must make healthy choices in your daily diet. If you are looking to maintain ideal body weight or you need to lose excess weight, you need to cut your carbohydrate intake, while taking enough protein to preserve muscle mass. Include anti-inflammatory foods, anti-oxidants, and polyflavonoids in your diet to manage chronic pain.

To follow a successful dietary pattern, RELATE FOOD TO FUEL RATHER THAN TO PLEASURE. Moreover, ensure that your diet plan is sustainable in the long run. It should be feasible for you to follow. Our nutritionists at Alleviate will help with tailor-made diet plans specific to your conditions.

Precepts and Precautions

1. What you eat matters: A balanced diet is essential for a healthy life
2. You cannot run for long on empty
3. Keep your energy bank charged
4. Persistent nutrient deficiency leads to chronic ailments

5. Supplements and superfoods are not a myth
6. Ideal body weight takes a load off your joints
7. Keep yourself hydrated

12

CLINICAL PSYCHOLOGY: THE LAW OF ATTRACTION

"If You can change your mind, You can change your life."
— William James

Everyone likes to associate with people who are upbeat and enthusiastic about life. Have you wondered why this is so? People who exude a positive attitude generally have a positive self-image. This allows them to be confident in themselves and assertive. This frame of mind leads to a healthy and happy life. In fact, many experts say that there is a link between positivity and good health. Optimistic or positive-minded people keep their focus on what they want in life and keep looking for ways to achieve their goals. These goals may be related to their education, work, physical health, relationships, etc. They have the confidence that they will definitely reach whatever goal they aim for.

Even when they face a problem or a difficulty along the way, or things do not go as they hoped for, they still look for something beneficial or good in the situation.

Think Positive

You may be now thinking, how is positivity or positive thinking related to chronic pain. Let me tell you a story. Manu and Suri were two boys who lived in a village. Manu was six years old and Suri was eight. They were very good friends and would always be found in each other's company. Although they were in different classes in the village school, the minute the final period ended, they would rush out of the school compound together, planning what games they would play that evening.

Soon, it was summer, and the school closed for a long vacation. The two friends now had all day to play and enjoy themselves. They usually stayed in the vicinity of their village, but one fine morning they were so intent on chasing some pretty butterflies that without their knowledge they went quite far from their village. Still, it was a beautiful day, and they were quite taken up by their surroundings. There were so many new things to discover and new places to explore. As they were prancing around the fields far from home, Manu suddenly heard a loud cry of distress. He quickly looked around, but could not find his friend anywhere. Suri had fallen into an open well. He did not know how to swim and in panic, he shouted out again. Manu ran to the well and looked down. He saw his friend struggling at the bottom.

He quickly looked around and spotted a big bucket with a rope attached. He picked it up and let the bucket down into the well. "Do not be afraid. Climb into the bucket and I will pull you up," he reassured Suri. As soon as the bucket hit the bottom, Suri got in. Manu felt the rope tug in his hands, and he started pulling up the bucket. It was difficult and his small hands were aching, but he did not stop pulling the rope. He was intent on saving his friend's life. The bucket slowly inched up and soon reached the top. Suri jumped out and both the friends hugged each other, and now both of them were wet. The boys quickly ran home and all the villagers were astonished to see both the boys soaked to their skins. However, when they heard the story of Suri's rescue, they did not believe it.

"Impossible," they said. "Manu is too young to pull up a bucket with a boy out of the well. He can barely lift a bucket of water, as it is." Both the boys insisted that it was true. "It simply is not possible," they said.

Even as this argument was going on, Ramu Kaka gestured with his hand for silence. Ramu Kaka was a wise elder of the village and people respected his words greatly. "I believe you both," he said. "But Ramu Kaka, he is not strong enough. How could he have done it?" everybody shouted. "Just as he mentioned. He pulled Suri up in a bucket," said Ramu Kaka.

Seeing the disbelieving faces all around, Ramu Kaka continued, "Let me explain. When Manu realized that Suri's life was in danger, his one thought was to rescue him. He did not pause to consider whether he had the strength. He just decided to do something and did it. There was no one around either to discourage him or tell him that it was an impossible task for him! If you believe you can do something, you definitely will succeed."

Believe and You Can Do It

The same holds true for any situation in life. What you believe is important. Your beliefs, whether positive or negative, determine what you do in life. When it comes to chronic pain, we have seen in the previous chapters, the various ways of managing the same. However, I have stressed the importance of a multidisciplinary approach in all the chapters. The multidisciplinary approach to managing chronic pain includes lifestyle changes as well, such as weight loss, regular exercise, proper nutritional intake, good control of blood sugar levels in a diabetic, and many others. Although medical professionals can help guide one in this process, the major effort has to be from the patient's side.

The patient must want to get well. Whatever treatment is given, the result depends finally on the patient's mindset. Simply stated, unless your mind is geared toward getting better, you will not see the expected result. This means you should be willing to make a change.

I have seen this widely in my clinical practice. The same treatment and advice may be meted out to 10 patients, but the ones who generally get better are those with a positive mindset. They follow the multidisciplinary approach that has been planned for them to the letter. They are careful about their nutritional intake, diligent in exercising daily, perform muscle-strengthening exercises regularly, and are careful about their weight gain. These people have a positive outlook in general.

Your mind is a powerful entity. You can change your life when you fill your mind with positive thoughts. If you want to change your body, you first have to change your mind.

There is great power in positive thinking. Tony Robbins, the American speaker and self-help coach, puts it like this: *"Whatever you hold in your mind on a consistent basis is exactly what you will experience in your life."* Your mindset controls your life. If you cannot control your mind, that means you cannot control your actions. You cannot succeed in following a disciplined lifestyle. For a better life, it is absolutely essential that you change your mindset and control your mind. Only then can you come out of the destructive cycle or lifestyle practices that are holding you back.

This is not a difficult thing to do. You just must want to get better and decide, 'Come what may, I will stick to the plan and follow it.'

I always tell my patients this: WHAT YOU SINCERELY THINK ABOUT, ARDENTLY WISH FOR, AND DESIRE WHOLEHEARTEDLY, YOU WILL GET. The keyword here is 'SINCERELY,' for as we all are aware, just plain wishful thinking will get one nowhere.

So, how can one become a person with a positive mindset? Somebody who has been suffering from pain for a long time is likely to say, "I don't think I will ever recover from this disease that is causing me pain.

I have lived with it for so long. I have consulted many health professionals and yet obtained no relief. I think I will have to live with the pain all my life." This is a wrong belief. Thinking this way will only hinder your recovery.

To start with, you must have a strong belief system. It can be your belief in God, belief in the medical profession and treatment, or just a belief in yourself. That is the first step. Theodore Roosevelt said, *"Believe you can, and you are halfway there."* You must believe in your potential, your strength, your skills, your decisions, and your intelligence.

In my practice, I have seen repeatedly that only the believers tend to get better with treatment and generally do well. The non-believers are non-starters. Why do I say that? The case study given below will help you understand the importance of a positive mindset and belief in oneself.

CASE STUDY 22

Sidharth was a 58-year-old software engineer working with an MNC in Bangalore. He came to our clinic with severe low back pain. He gave a history of having had this pain for the past 10 years. He had undergone a fusion procedure in the back on the advice of his orthopedic surgeon about four years ago. While initially there was some relief, the pain recurred. As the years passed, the pain was becoming more intense and was seriously hampering his quality of life. On examination we found him to be obese. He had been leading a sedentary lifestyle with almost no physical exercise. His work involved sitting in one place for long periods in an AC room. He hardly moved out of his office during his workday. His eating habits were not very healthy either. He did not have his meals at regular times. He also used to eat a lot of junk food.

After assessing him completely at Alleviate, we advised him about adopting lifestyle changes in addition to regenerative therapy for pain relief. Sidharth was very receptive to all the suggestions.

He made an effort to understand all the different facets of the multidisciplinary approach that we were explaining to him.

He showed eagerness to begin the treatment and was decisive about doing his part. He underwent five to six sessions of PrP plus Prolotherapy for lower back strengthening. He was diligent in following the entire treatment plan as per schedule. He visited Alleviate for three months of extensive physical therapy sessions. Following these sessions, he continued physiotherapy regularly at home as well. He was serious about losing the excess weight and followed the dietary advice given by our in-house nutritionist. He followed the diet chart carefully. He ensured that he got some exercise at least five days a week. He took to walking and also joined an online Yoga class. Overall, he approached his treatment with a lot of positivity and hence was able to stick to the plan. He was able to achieve what he set out to do.

Now three years later, he is feeling much better. There is no back pain. He has lost a substantial amount of weight, which has made him a much more confident person. He was an avid golfer in his younger days and now he has returned to the game with gusto. He is able to travel to different places to play golf. He loves spending time with his two grandchildren, running around, and playing active games with them.

Now let me tell you about Ankit.

Ankit was a 54-year-old executive in an IT firm. He came to see us at Alleviate with a similar complaint: persistent low back pain. Ankit too had been having the pain for a number of years and had undergone a spinal fusion procedure, which failed to relieve his pain.

His history too was similar to Sidharth's. On examination, he was extremely obese and had difficulty walking. He too was following a sedentary lifestyle with almost no physical exercise. His work too involved sitting in one room for long periods. He too did not have healthy eating habits.

However, the one difference here was in the attitude. Whereas Sidharth had a positive outlook and was willing to wholeheartedly try to change his life, Ankit had a very negative approach.

He suffered from low self-esteem. He was given the same advice about lifestyle modification and following the multidisciplinary approach. But he was not very receptive to these ideas. He would say, "What's the use of anything? I cannot exercise. How will I lose weight? It is impossible for me. Just give me some treatment for relief from this back pain." He did not make any attempt to understand or follow the different features of the multidisciplinary approach despite our assurances that we would help him. He too underwent around five sessions of PrP plus Prolotherapy for the back pain. However, he was adamant in his belief that it was impossible for him to make any lifestyle changes. He lost all motivation and soon developed an eating disorder.

Three years later, he became morbidly obese, which is a life-threatening condition. He was admitted and was lying on the operation theater table waiting for a life-saving bariatric surgical procedure. You can see how his life had spiraled downhill. Now, these are two people who came with the same complaint—failed back surgery for low back pain. Their problems were similar—both were overweight—and their jobs and lifestyles were similar too. Both of them were required to make lifestyle modifications with regard to diet, exercise, physiotherapy, etc.

However, the difference lay in their psychology. One person approached his problem with a positive attitude. The other person viewed his situation negatively and was not even willing to make an effort in the right direction. He thought it to be hopeless. That is why I say, non-believers are non-starters. Only if you believe that you can achieve something, will you even take the first step toward it.

The First Step Toward Change/Banish Negativity

Accept that you need to make a change to better your life.

It may be with regard to dieting, weight loss, or following a regular exercise schedule, or any other lifestyle modification. The first crucial step is to accept the need to change. Next, you have to believe it is possible to achieve it. If you start with doubts and a feeling of hopelessness, then you cannot succeed. Negative thoughts can strangle your self-confidence. Bikram Chaudhary, the renowned Yoga guru, says thus: *"Negative attitude is nine times more powerful than positive attitude."* This will give you an idea of how dangerous it is to harbor a negative attitude toward your health.

In the management of chronic pain, along with specific targeted therapy, general good health is a requisite. You must take control of your life. Do not speak negative words about yourself. Words are known to have power and energy. Change how you speak about yourself and your problems. Do not let negative thoughts hold you back. Do not become your own enemy. Do not put a limit on your abilities. *"Negative thinking definitely attracts negative results"*—Norman Vincent Peale. On the other hand, a positive attitude can definitely help you achieve your goal. When you speak out something aloud, you are the first person to hear it. So, make sure you are speaking out the right things, positive things.

Think 'I Can'/The Law of Attraction

Have an attitude of 'I can'. Having a positive attitude or thoughts attracts positive outcomes and events. This is the law of attraction. When you have a positive attitude and also put in your diligent effort, you will definitely see results. When you have a positive attitude and put in your best effort you will be able to get over any hindrances and slowly and surely move toward your goal.

However, much others may encourage you, the effort has to come from you. Only you can empower yourself with the important weapon of self-confidence, which is necessary when you are setting out to change your life.

It requires courage and determination.

You may fail a time or two. Maybe you were not able to keep to your exercise schedule or you cheated on your diet. Do not let this deter you. Reset your goals and keep trying. So far, I have talked about making a physical change or a lifestyle change to make you healthy and thereby aid in reducing pain. Let us now talk about the psychological aspect.

The Psychology of Pain

Apart from the medical treatment for pain, which includes medication, surgery, and physical therapy, psychological therapy also plays an important role in pain management. Chronic pain is a stressful condition, and stress can lead to other problems in the body, such as high blood pressure, heart disease, obesity, diabetes, and depression. So, it is essential that one should learn how to cope with stress. Pain can also be compounded by stress or anxiety. The psychologist can help you with coping techniques. They will talk to you and find out things that are causing you worry or anxiety. They will discuss what causes stress in your life. What are the causes that increase your pain?

Psychologists tell us that in chronic pain, apart from the pain per se, emotional and psychological factors play a significant role as well. A patient suffering from chronic pain might be experiencing feelings of anger, anxiety, hopelessness, despair, etc.

Psychologists can help you understand your thoughts, emotions, and behavior. They will create or design a treatment plan specific to the patient, which can include teaching a relaxation technique or changing your beliefs about your pain. They will teach you techniques to distract yourself from the pain or sleep techniques to help you sleep better. Managing stress can help relieve pain to a great extent.

Psychologists can also help you make the lifestyle changes that are necessary for you. Basically, you will be taught to develop skills to cope with your pain. Pain psychologists provide psychological therapy in conjunction with medical therapy.

That is, even as you are being treated by your doctor for pain with medicines or regenerative therapy or physiotherapy, you can take the help of the clinical psychologist as well.

We provide clinical psychology counseling to all our patients who are suffering from chronic pain. The psychologist can help devise adaptive strategies and reduce the emotional distress in the patient. They can help foster positive thoughts and beliefs.

Psychological therapy may be given as individual counseling or family counseling, as the case requires. This is termed cognitive behavioral therapy (CBT). This involves imparting the following skills to the patient:

- General stress management
- Relaxation techniques
- Health promotion
- Anger management
- Understanding oneself
- Activity pacing
- Acceptance and awareness
- Adaptive behaviors
- Combating clinical depression and anxiety
- Fostering a positive outlook

Here is what Ms. Sonam Manoj, the clinical psychologist at Alleviate has to say about the role of health and clinical psychology in chronic pain management.

Scene: *The patient is sitting on a chair opposite the therapist. He appears to be uncomfortable and keeps shifting and fidgeting in his seat. He gives the impression of being distressed and a little bit confused as well.*

Patient: *I want to start by clarifying that I am not faking my pain, or manifesting pain. My pain is real. I am not hallucinating, and I am not mad.*

Therapist: *I believe you. I understand that you are in pain. I believe that the pain is real and you are not faking it. However, let us work together and find out how you can feel better. We need to discover what is increasing your pain and also what can decrease it.*

Here, the psychologist plays a part of non-judgmentally listening to the patient and giving him/her the reassurance that indeed the feeling of pain is true and existent. The factors that play a role in increasing or alleviating the pain experience need to be explained to the patient. Awareness is provided to the patient in terms of the psychosocial factors that play a role in the pain challenges.

This is a common picture of the first meeting of a patient suffering from chronic pain with a pain psychologist. This scenario will give you a general idea of how a patient experiencing chronic pain thinks. He/she probably thinks that people do not believe them. It is very important to reassure them that we do not doubt the validity of their distress. As research has increasingly made clear the physiological basis of pain and the different receptors and mechanisms that are at play, the scope of a psychologist in the field of pain management has evolved as well. In recent times, the role of the mind in pain perception and the relevance of 'mind and its play' has been studied extensively, and there is still a lot more to be discovered.

Clinical and health psychologists have been looking closely at the psychosocial factors involved in the treatment and management of chronic pain and this deeper study has helped them improve the biopsychosocial framework for chronic pain management.

In the present time, clinical and health psychology has helped by providing protocols, evidence, treatment, and solutions in different fields of medical science—psycho-oncology, psychocardiology, neuropsychology, and pain psychology. About 14 percent of the disease burden in the world has been attributed to neuropsychiatric disorders, mainly owing to the chronic nature of these illnesses.

In their article titled "*No health without mental health*" in *The Lancet*, Prince et al.[6] have said that having many diseases or comorbidities increases the chances of the patient being in poor mental health.

In the field of pain management, it is important to remember that there is a bidirectional relationship between chronic pain and anxiety or depression.

When a person with depression undergoes pain for a long time, it has been observed that the brain can combine the two experiences. This makes it difficult for the patient to differentiate the two experiences as separate. Patients suffering from depression or anxiety disorders often complain about physical pain as well.

Similarly, when one is going through a phase of chronic pain, the associated immobility experienced can add to the difficulties in their activities of daily living. It can increase the dysfunctionality in daily life experienced by the patient. This can further affect the person's self-regard and self-esteem and lead to their having anxiety-causing moments, distress, and episodes of depression. It can be described as a chain reaction.

Pain psychologists have much to offer in these situations, and seeking their help when going through chronic pain is always a great and informed decision. Numerous clinical trials have been conducted in the field of pain psychology that have helped to formulate different approaches to understanding and managing the emotions, thought processes, and behaviors that usually occur as by-products or effects of chronic pain. The aim of pain psychology is to reduce the patient's inflexibility toward their pain and assist them in making their quality of life better. Clinical psychology in pain management has contributed enormously toward framing guidelines and best practices for more efficacious implementation of treatments and protocols.

---

[6]https://pubmed.ncbi.nlm.nih.gov/17804063/

CASE STUDY 23

Gita is a 37-year-old former tech executive who came to our clinic with a history of back pain radiating to her right leg for the past eight years. She also presented with allodynia and hyperalgesia. In allodynia, there is increased pain and sensitivity to even mild stimuli such as touch, and hyperalgesia, as the name suggests, means having an increased sensitivity to pain. On neurological examination, there was no abnormality detected in her motor system and all her reflexes were normal. However, the straight leg raising test was restricted to 30 degrees in both legs because of pain. She mentions during her evaluation that she was 'just fine' until she got injured on the job around eight years ago. Due to the increasing severity of the pain, she was forced to resign from her job. Now she just sits at home for most of her days, despite her husband's attempts to get her out of the house and take a walk with him. She avoids going out of the house because she is worried about getting pain flare-ups. She feels that if she experienced a pain flare-up, she would immediately want to lie down to alleviate the pain, and this would be impossible if she was outdoors at that time. She fears being judged by the people around her if she had to ask for help in public. She avoids going to all social and family gatherings because she feels she is not as brisk and quick as the others of her age are. She fears being termed as a sick or lethargic person.

Depression and Anxiety Scale (HADS). However, she denies having any suicidal thoughts. At home, she often broods over her life and focuses on all that she has lost over the years, especially her job loss. She imagines a future where she is housebound, dependent, neglected, and lonely. Often, in this frame of mind, she becomes short-tempered and snaps at her daughter or says mean things to her husband. She later regrets her words and dissolves into tears.

She underwent a psychological evaluation and scored high for depression on the Hospital Depression And Anxiety Scale (HDAS). So, how would a clinical psychologist help this patient? In such a situation, the typical interventions by a psychologist would be the following:

1. CBT for chronic pain where the patient is taught to make small changes in their learned helpless behavior. The patient is encouraged to change or avoid saying sentences such as "I will need help because I am definitely going to have a flare-up if I go out of the house," "I am not healthy as I was before," "I cannot work by myself or look after myself anymore."

2. Acceptance and commitment therapy (ACT): Here the patient is taught to defuse or dissociate from the thought of pain. The aim here is to make them understand this concept: I am not pain; pain is not me. Next, they are led to take committed action toward the goal of becoming functional again. The patient, in the end, is able to accept the situation the way it is. ACT is a well-researched intervention in the field of pain psychology.

3. Guided imagery: This is a low-cost but effective way to reduce pain signals and enhance pain tolerance. The patient is taught to relax and envision a better and pain-free future in her mind.

4. Multidisciplinary interventions by trained paramedics to address all the other concerns as well. The biopsychosocial approach addresses all the elements involved in the patient's illness.

In short, clinical psychology can help decipher the psychological make-up of patients suffering from chronic pain, such as the co-existence of anxiety or depression, the inflexible attitude of the patient to his/her situation, or acceptance of the situation by the patient.

This knowledge lets the pain psychologist work on the patient's belief system and expectations, and identify the placebo and nocebo effects. They can thus help the patient cope better with their pain symptoms and lead a more functional life than they would have done otherwise. Thus, you can see there is help out there for managing chronic pain. You do not have to do it alone. You just have to set your mind to do whatever it takes. Take the first step. Come see us at Alleviate and our clinical psychologist will definitely help you.

Precepts and Precautions

1. Be positive/believe in yourself
2. Challenge yourself to make a change and try new things
3. Be patient and trust your journey
4. Keep trying until you reach your target
5. Seek professional help for mind and body
6. Remember success depends on your attitude, commitment, and self-discipline

13

THE ALLEVIATE WAY

Control your destiny—Be empowered to make a change

Dear reader, we are now almost at the end of this book. I have endeavored to present the various conditions that can possibly result in chronic pain and the different treatment methods and options available for managing the same. In this chapter, I wish to stress the Alleviate Way to managing chronic pain. As you read through the previous chapters of this book, you are bound to have come across the term MULTIDISCIPLINARY APPROACH.

To state it in simple terms, the Alleviate Way is the Multidisciplinary Approach that we follow. In fact, the multidisciplinary approach is one of the elements of our Mission Statement. It is the cornerstone of our treatment protocols.

What is this Multidisciplinary Approach?

As the term suggests, a multidisciplinary approach basically

209

means that different members of the healthcare team or different specialists care for the patient, seeing to all his health needs simultaneously.

How does this approach impact a patient's health and healing?

To make this clear, I would like to bring in the analogy of a plant again. A sapling growing in a plant bed has numerous requirements to grow into a healthy plant. It requires good soil with appropriate nutrients, adequate exposure to sunlight, enough water content in the soil, favorable weather conditions, and the care and concern of the gardener. All these factors aid the sapling in growing into a strong robust plant or tree.

When the sapling first germinated, the conditions of the soil might have been just right. However, for the plant to continue to grow in a healthy way, it is important that these optimum conditions are maintained. Even as the plant is growing, it might be exposed to numerous adverse conditions, such as bad climate, drought, extreme weather conditions, or nutrient-depleted soil. When the gardener comes across a plant that is not healthy, he does not just water the plant or position the plant away from the direct rays of the sun. He makes a comprehensive check first to identify all the factors that need to be rectified. He then institutes all the changes and only then does the plant regain its health. The same holds true for the human body as well. When young children are still being cared for by their parents, they receive optimal nurturing. Their physical and emotional needs are adequately met. They get enough exercise as they run around and play. They are taught other life skills as well, such as communication. The parents ensure that their children get timely and adequate food and rest. However, as adults, we rarely take care of ourselves so well. Owing to faulty lifestyle patterns, faulty eating habits, and faulty sleep patterns we fall prey to a lot of diseases.

Now to manage these disease conditions, we consult doctors or specialists who treat the individual problems.

At Alleviate, our message to patients is this: Along with getting treatment for your primary condition, it is also important to ensure that all other factors that play a role in keeping you healthy are in optimal condition as well. Results from any treatment can be optimized and sustained only when the patient is healthy in all aspects. This may be with regard to their weight, eating habits, sleep pattern, mental and emotional state, or physical exercise.

All these factors have to be in harmony, and function well for the patient to be restored to good health. The WHO definition of health states health to be "a complete physical, mental, and social wellbeing and not merely the absence of disease or infirmity." The WHO's call for the total well-being of the patient translates directly to the multidisciplinary approach when dealing with any illness.

At Alleviate, we have found the multidisciplinary approach to be definitely far better for healing chronic painful conditions than the single-specialty input method. In fact, we encourage our patients to believe that for good physical health and sustained pain relief, it is essential that multiple aspects of their body and lifestyle are functioning optimally. If they are not, then they need to be set right along with the specific treatment for their condition.

To help you better understand how the multidisciplinary approach to chronic pain helps patients, I would like to discuss a couple of conditions that we have already seen in the previous chapters. Fibromyalgia and chronic low back pain are two conditions that can have quite a debilitating effect on patients.

These are two conditions that can not only curtail the quality of life of the affected person but also extract an emotional toll from them.

Condition 1: Fibromyalgia

In the chapter on fibromyalgia, you would have read about Latha Seshadri, a 47-year-old college professor.

When she came to Alleviate with a long history of chronic body pain, we diagnosed her to have fibromyalgia.

Latha, a vivacious and lively person, who immersed herself

wholeheartedly in whatever activity she was involved in, had become a moody, depressed person by the time of her diagnosis.

She was unable to perform her daily activities of living and her quality of life had diminished to a great extent. She was also found to be mildly overweight and had mild hypertension as well.

The multidisciplinary approach followed in Alleviate helped Latha enormously in dealing with her condition. She was given trigger point injection therapy and physiotherapy to manage the symptoms of fibromyalgia.

Apart from that, the lifestyle consultant was able to help Latha in planning a daily routine that she would be comfortable following. The clinical nutritionist prepared tailor-made diet plans specifically to cater to her requirements. The clinical counseling provided to her and her family members went a long way in educating them about the nature of Latha's ailment and the different resources that were available to them. Counseling also gave the family insight into Latha's mindset and opened up the possible ways in which they could be supportive of her.

We have already learned that fibromyalgia is a condition that presents with symptoms of pain in various areas of the body but with no specific external physical signs. This makes the diagnosis of the disease particularly challenging. In fact, we can say that 70 percent of medical practitioners would not be aware of the incidence and symptoms of fibromyalgia in the community they are practicing in.

When patients present with long-standing nonspecific chronic pain, they are often told that nothing is wrong with them and that they are probably imagining the pain. Diagnosing and treating a patient with fibromyalgia requires patience and time. At Alleviate, we take time to give the patient our whole attention. They are not made to feel hurried in any way. We allow the patient to feel that we are taking their complaints seriously and are going to look for ways to make them feel better.

This goes a long way in reassuring these patients, because till then most probably their pain would have been brushed off.

We explain to the patient that what we would be doing is the

STEP-UP approach to managing fibromyalgia. First, if they are not already receiving optimum treatment, we initiate treatment with pain medications. The patient is prescribed specific customized physical therapy sessions as well.

If the patient shows a good response to the pain with this therapy, it is continued. However, the symptoms may not be adequately controlled with this alone; in such cases, we move on or STEP-UP to trigger point injections and infusion treatments.

Along with these mainline therapies, the patients are given nutritional counseling and psychological counseling. They are taught ways in which they can manage their symptoms better. The family is given counseling as well so that they can be supportive of the patient.

We emphasize that no treatment or approach is more important when compared to another. All are equally important in the care of the fibromyalgia patient.

Having this kind of comprehensive encompassing care reassures the patient greatly and benefits them to a large extent by decreasing their pain and distress.

Condition 2: Chronic Low Back Pain

Again, looking at a patient from one of the earlier chapters—Chronic Pain Generators In The Spine—I would like to illustrate the role of the multidisciplinary approach in patient healing. Mrs. Murthy was an elderly lady who came to Alleviate with a longstanding history of back pain. She had been to multiple practitioners and tried various remedies over the years. Her condition had never been diagnosed accurately and the treatments had mainly been a hodgepodge of trial-and-error methods. In fact, she had even been advised to undergo a surgical procedure on the spine, which she did.

She underwent fusion surgery of the spine, which far from relieving her pain, actually resulted in increasing the severity of the back pain.

Lack of proper postsurgery rehabilitation and patient counseling resulted in her having failed back surgery syndrome.

When Mrs. Murthy came to Alleviate, she underwent a complete physical assessment. Based on imaging studies, she was diagnosed to have sacroiliac joint disease. She was also found to be slightly obese. Treatment for her condition was initiated immediately. As she had already been on various oral pain medications with no relief, we began treating her with anti-inflammatory injections. Following this, she underwent six sessions of Prolotherapy for the back spread across two months. She experienced immediate relief from pain. She underwent multiple sessions of physical therapy and was advised that this would need to be continued long-term. Her weight problem was also addressed. She was counseled by our nutritionist who helped her understand how being overweight could lead to a detrimental effect on her joints and actually result in chronic pain. She was prescribed a diet plan suitable for her. Our physical therapists also taught her simple exercises that she could follow at home. This concerted care by the whole team brought about a complete change in Mrs. Murthy. Not only was she relieved of her longstanding back pain, but also her quality of life changed for the better in all aspects. She became independent and mobile, and her frame of mind also improved. Where she used to be quite depressed about her pain and immobility, she now had a positive and happier outlook. This case highlights the importance of the multidisciplinary approach in dealing with chronic back pain. Chronic back pain cannot be attributed to a single cause, and therefore, the management of the same involves the resolving of multiple issues. For instance, people resort to self-medication when they experience back pain without getting it properly diagnosed by a doctor.Again, when patients are advised to undergo physical therapy, they may go for three or four sessions and then discontinue. Or when they do undergo back surgery, such as fusion of the spine, they do not follow any postsurgery rehabilitation measures. All these scenarios can be avoided with the multidisciplinary approach, where the patient is given adequate counseling and support in all these areas.

Proper counseling and guidance with postsurgical therapy can prevent patients from developing failed back surgery.

Facets of the Multidisciplinary Approach

1. Assessment: A complete assessment of the patient's health is made. This does not involve only the presenting complaint of the patient, but also their general mental and physical health. For example, patients may be assessed to find out if they are overweight, whether they have any comorbidities, such as hypertension and diabetes, if they are depressed, etc.

2. Diagnosis: A diagnosis of the patient's condition is arrived at after a complete physical examination and the required imaging studies are completed.

3. Pre-habilitation: This is where a patient is prepared both physically and mentally to receive the specified treatment. This increases the capacity of the patient to withstand medical or surgical therapy. For instance, if the patient is supposed to undergo a surgical procedure, pre-habilitation will help them with exercises to strengthen the back. It also helps patients begin their treatment with a positive mindset, which goes a long way in their recovery. Pre-habilitation also has a role to play in reducing the side effects of the medical or surgical interventions that the patients undergo.

4. Therapy: The treatment appropriate and custom-made for each patient is instituted by professionals trained in their respective fields. The timely and correct treatment brings about an early cure. Or else, it can help in preventing the worsening of the patient's condition. In many instances, at Alleviate, we are trying to prevent patients from reaching a stage where surgical management is inevitable.

5. Rehabilitation: The patients are taught about the follow-up measures they have to follow once they have completed their specified therapy. It may be coming in for regular sessions of physical therapy. Or it may involve following a

weight-loss diet regimen. Post-therapy rehabilitation is very important in a patient's recovery. Patients are taught how they can optimize their lifestyle to get maximum benefits from the therapy.

6. Counseling: In many instances, both patients and their family members benefit from counseling. The importance of taking small steps on a consistent basis is explained to the patient. The family members too need to be informed about the care and support that they can extend to the patient on their road to recovery. Encouragement and support of the family members play a major role in keeping patients in a positive mindset.

Therefore, it follows that the multidisciplinary approach will involve team members from various disciplines. It is an integrated team approach to patient care where all the members of the health team structure and deliver patient-centered treatments and share the responsibility as well.

Resources at Alleviate

Our Professionals:

At Alleviate, we have a dedicated team of doctors and specialists who uphold the multidisciplinary approach to manage patients with chronic pain. We have orthopedic surgeons, specialists trained in critical care and pain medicine, specialists in spine surgery, specialists in anesthesia and interventional pain management, diabetologists, and lifestyle consultants on our staff. Our physiotherapists are specially trained and skilled in sports and neurorehabilitation. They can prescribe custom-made exercise therapies for patients.

They are experienced in procedures such as fascia release, soft tissue release, dry needling, and manual therapy. We also have on our staff a clinical nutrition expert who can guide our patients ably in their nutritional and diet requirements. Our clinical psychologists help patients and their relatives through their counseling sessions. They are trained in pain psychology and can tailor therapies for patients suffering from fibromyalgia, stress-related pain, etc.

Chronic Pain Conditions Treated:

At Alleviate, we treat the following pain conditions after diagnosing the underlying disease with the help of a thorough history, detailed clinical examination, and relevant investigations.
- Knee pain
- Back pain
- Shoulder pain
- Neck pain
- Foot and ankle pain
- Hand and wrist pain
- Fibromyalgia
- Headache and migraine
- Trigger points
- Cancer pain

Facilities/Procedures:

The various procedures and treatment methods available at Alleviate are listed below:
- Stem Cell Therapy
- Platelet Rich Plasma (ISO approved)
- Prolotherapy
- Radiofrequency Ablation
- Cooled Radiofrequency Ablation (US FDA approved)
- Image-guided Needle-based Interventions
- Viscosupplementation
- Steroid Injections
- Endoscopic Spine Surgery

- Image-guided Nerve Blocks
- BOTOX Injections
- Intravenous Infusions

Our Treatment Protocols:

1. We follow the complete allopathic approach to pain management.
2. We follow the multidisciplinary approach to treat chronic pain.
3. Doctor-led clinical management.
4. Precise image-guided procedures (Fluoroscopy and Ultrasound).

Benefits of the Multidisciplinary Approach

1. The patient is looked at as a whole and all his/her needs are identified.
2. The patient is provided the required pre-habilitation, which readies them for the medical, surgical, or interventional treatment that they will be undergoing.
3. Treatment regimens can be tailor-made for each patient taking their individual requirements into consideration.
4. The results of treatment are found to be better and sustained.
5. Patient satisfaction is increased when all their problems are taken note of.
6. Emotional and mental health is given importance. Both these factors play a crucial role in the well-being of the patient.
7. It helps empower the patient, thereby allowing them to set targets and goals in their journey to recovery.

The Alleviate Way

In short, The Alleviate Way may be summarized as following these principles:

(A) Empathy and Patience: The patient is looked at as a whole person. We take the time to assess not just the physical condition, but also to find out all that is on their mind. We look at the different ways in which we can help them.

(B) Education of the Patient: We firmly believe that an educated patient is an empowered patient. We help our patients understand their illnesses. This goes a long way in helping our patients cope with their illness and also patient compliance to the treatment.

(C) Multidisciplinary Approach: This is the cornerstone of our treatment strategy. Our patients have benefitted enormously and experienced excellent relief from chronic pain as a result of this methodology.

(D) Patient Participation: We encourage patient participation in the treatment strategies. A patient who is aware and knowledgeable about his/her health condition can actively participate in all the treatment methods, thereby resulting in an optimal effect.

(E) Focus on Quality of Life: We focus not just on the temporary relief of pain but on improving the Quality of Life of the patient.

14

SYMPTOMATOLOGY OF COMMON CONDITIONS CAUSING CHRONIC PAIN

Know your symptoms: The first step to a diagnosis

Having read through this book, you would have come across the myriad conditions that can cause chronic pain. You would also have read about all the numerous other symptoms that can accompany these conditions. I have endeavored in the preceding chapters to present a comprehensive compendium of all the conditions that can result in chronic pain.

For most people, a particular chapter may be relevant to their pain or a loved one's condition. Or at the most, maybe two chapters. Now here, in this chapter, I present an easy symptom guide that will help you identify the cause of chronic pain quickly. Are your symptoms confusing you? At times you may not be sure of how to address your pain symptoms. This symptom guide will help resolve the confusion. Once you know what you are likely suffering from, the next step to treatment is quite easy.

Common Conditions Affecting the Neck

Cervical Radiculopathy
- Sharp, electric-shock-like pain, radiating down from the neck, along the shoulder, into the arm, hand, and fingers.
- Tingling, numbness, and weakness in the arms and hands.
- Symptoms described as the feeling of pins and needles.
- Difficulty experienced in routine activities such as typing, holding objects, and getting dressed.
- Pain due to disc involvement (discogenic pain) is usually aggravated by neck movements and relieved by rest.

Cervical Facet Syndrome
- Symptoms can range from occasional discomfort to severe persistent pain
- Can seriously affect the quality of life.
- In the early stages, there may be stiffness and dull ache rather than sharp pain.
- Onset of pain is gradual, and it slowly progresses over time.
- Rest can help relieve pain flare-ups.
- Pain can radiate to the shoulder on one side or between the shoulder blades.
- Pressing down on the neck can elicit pain.
- Pain and stiffness are more pronounced in the mornings, and may reduce in intensity as the day progresses.
- Pain may be aggravated at the end of the day.
- Advanced stages can have continuous pain that disturbs the person's sleep as well.
- Headache may be present, usually in the back of the head.

Common Conditions Affecting the Shoulders

Frozen Shoulder

- The shoulder capsule becomes thick and stiff, leading to severe pain and inability to move the shoulder.
- There are three stages to the condition.

   Stage 1: Freezing. There is a worsening of pain and a decrease in the range of movements. This stage can last from 6 weeks to 9 months.

   Stage 2: Frozen. There may be a decrease in the pain symptoms, but the joint stiffness remains. This stage can last 4 months to 6 months. The patient may find it difficult to perform daily activities of living.

   Stage 3: Thawing. There is a slow improvement of the shoulder movements at this stage. It can take anywhere from 6 months to 2 years for the return of normal strength and movements in the affected shoulder.

Rotator Cuff Injuries

- These injuries can be caused by either acute tears or degenerative tears.
- Patients may experience pain at rest during the night, especially if they sleep on the affected side.
- Pain may be felt while lifting or lowering the arm on the affected side. Or the pain may be felt with some other specific movements.
- Inability or difficulty in using the arm on the affected side to reach behind the back.
- There may be a progressive weakness when lifting or rotating the arm on the affected side.
- Moving the shoulder may result in crepitus or a crackling sensation.

Common Conditions Affecting the Back and Spine

Sacroiliac Joint Dysfunction

- Lower back pain: Below the level of L5 vertebra.
- Pain, numbness, tingling, and weakness may be felt in the lower extremity.
- Pain may be present in the pelvis or buttocks regions.
- Pain can spread to the hip/groin area.
- Stiffness and reduced range of movement in the lower back, hips, pelvis, and groin.
- The pain worsens on climbing stairs, running, jogging, etc.
- Leg instability: buckling or giving way of the leg while walking.
- Pain causes disturbance in sleep.
- Inability to sit for prolonged periods of time.
- Pain on moving from sitting to standing position.

Facet Joint Syndrome

- Low back pain that has a deep dull aching character.
- Pain limited to the back and buttocks region.
- Pain is aggravated by standing for a long time.
- Early morning stiffness may be present.
- Pain is relieved by bending forward: the hunched position.
- Involvement of cervical and thoracic vertebrae can cause pain and stiffness in the neck, shoulders, and upper and mid-back regions.

Spondylolisthesis

- People with mild spondylolisthesis may not have any symptoms.
- Persistent lower back pain. Pain is worse when active or standing, and is relieved by lying down.
- Stiffness in the back and legs.

- Pain in the thighs.
- Tightening of the hamstrings and buttock muscles.
- Curvature of the spine in severe cases.
- Pain, numbness, or tingling spreading from the lower back down the legs (sciatica).

Failed Back Surgery

- Patients continue to experience pain even after undergoing spine surgery.
- Diffuse, dull, and aching pain involving the back or legs.
- Some patients may experience sharp pricking, burning, or stabbing pain in the extremities.

Piriformis Syndrome

- Acute tenderness in the buttock region and sciatica-like pain that radiates down the back of the thigh, calf, and foot.
- Dull ache in the buttock.
- Pain when walking upstairs or walking up an incline.
- Pain is increased after prolonged sitting.
- The hip joint exhibits a reduced range of movements.
- Pain can lessen on lying down, bending the knee, or walking.
- Patients may be seen to hold the affected buttock higher up while sitting.

Coccydynia

- There may be an aching or piercing pain in the tailbone area.
- Moving from sitting to a standing position can increase the severity of pain.
- Sitting for long periods of time can increase the severity of the pain.
- Pain during bowel movements.
- Pain during sex.
- Aching sensation in the buttocks.

Common Conditions Affecting the Knee

Arthritis Knee

- Pain in the affected knee joint.
- Swelling in the joint.
- Pain and swelling may be worse in the morning.
- Crepitations may be present in the affected joint.
- Grinding sensation may be felt in severe cases.
- Joint movements may be reduced.
- Joint tenderness and surrounding muscle tenderness may be present.
- There will be a loss of muscle strength.

Chondromalacia Patella

- Dull aching pain felt below the knee cap.
- Pain may be felt on the sides of the knee cap.
- Grinding sensation may be felt when the knee is flexed.
- The same sensation is present when going downstairs or running downhill.
- Grinding sensation felt when standing up after sitting down for a while.
- Mild swelling of the knee joint.

Ligament Injuries Related to Sports

- There are many ligaments in the knee joint that can be affected isolated or in combination.
- This can result in structural weakness in the affected knee joint.
- Patients can have difficulty in weight-bearing.
- Pain can be present during athletic activities.
- Early signs of degeneration can be present in the joint.

Bursitis

- Inflammation of a bursa in the knee joint.
- Affected portion of the knee feels warm, tender, and swollen.
- Pain may be present on moving the joint or at rest.
- Pain begins gradually and worsens over time.
- Commonly occurs in people who kneel for prolonged periods in their jobs.

Meniscus Tears

- Most common cartilage injury of the knee joint.
- Pain in the knee joint. Swelling in the affected knee.
- Popping sensation during the injury.
- Difficulty in bending and straightening the leg on the affected side.
- The affected knee joint tends to get 'locked' or 'stuck.'
- Decreased range of motion on the affected side.

Iliotibial Band Syndrome

- Inflammation of the iliotibial band where it moves back and forth across the femoral epicondyle.
- Initially stinging or needle-like pains are present.
- Pain on the lateral side of the knee.
- Pain progresses gradually and can become quite disabling.
- Pain can cause difficulty in walking or climbing upstairs and downstairs.
- Snapping or popping sounds may occur at the affected knee joint.
- Swelling may be present where the iliotibial band crosses the femoral epicondyle.
- Swelling may be present below the knee.
- Pain can radiate along the course of the iliotibial band along the outer side of the thigh till the hip.

Common Conditions Affecting the Elbow, Hand, and Wrist

Golfer's Elbow (Medial Epicondylitis)
- Inflammation of the tendons that connect the forearm to the elbow.
- Stiffness of the elbow joint is present.
- Pain and tenderness are present on the inner side of the elbow or the forearm.
- Pain when you try to make a fist on the affected side.
- Tingling and numbness may be present in the ring finger and the little finger.
- Weakness may be experienced in the hand and the wrist. Grip strength is decreased.

Tennis Elbow (Lateral Epicondylitis)
- Pain and tenderness can be present on the outer side of the elbow over the bony knob.
- Pain may radiate into the upper or lower arm.
- Pain can be manifest when you lift an object.
- Pain can occur when you open a door or shake hands with someone.
- Pain can occur when you raise your hand or straighten your wrist.
- Swelling around the elbow joint externally.
- Redness around the affected elbow joint.

Carpal Tunnel Syndrome
- Compression of the median nerve at the wrist.
- Symptoms start gradually and worsen with time.
- Tingling or numbness felt in the fingers or hand. Symptoms may involve the thumb, index, middle, and ring fingers. The little finger is usually spared.
- Electric shock-like sensations can occur, which travel up your arm from the wrist.
- Symptoms commonly occur when holding an object such

as a mobile phone or newspaper in the hand on the affected side. Weakness may be experienced in the hand, resulting in the dropping of objects.

- Weakness caused by the involvement of muscles involved in the pincer grip of the thumb.

De Quervain's Tenosynovitis

- Condition involves the tendons present on the thumb side of the wrist joint.
- Pain near the base of the thumb.
- Swelling may be present near the base of the thumb.
- Difficulty in performing grasping and pinching movements involving the thumb and wrist.
- Movement of the thumb causes a 'sticking' or 'stop-and-go' sensation.
- Snapping or popping sensation may be felt in the wrist while moving the thumb.

Common Conditions Affecting the Foot and Ankle

Plantar Fasciitis

- Pain in the heel or the surrounding tissues.
- Increase in intensity of the pain is felt after exercising but not during the exercise.
- Pain is felt in the arch of the foot.
- Pain can be worse on getting up in the morning or on standing up after sitting for a long time.
- Swelling in the heel area.
- Pain can be present for many months.
- Tightness felt in the Achilles tendon.

Retrocalcaneal Bursitis

- The main symptom is heel pain, which is mainly felt on

putting pressure on the heel.

- There may be swelling around the heel area posteriorly.
- Pain on leaning back on the heel.
- Standing up on toes can aggravate the pain.
- Pain may be present in the calf muscles while walking or running.
- Flexing of the foot may give rise to a crackling sound.
- Stiffness and loss of movements in the heel joint.
- Warmth and redness may be present at the back of the heel.

Achilles Tendonitis

- There may be pain and stiffness along the Achilles tendon in the morning. Pain that is present along the tendon or in the back of the heel can worsen with activity.
- Severe pain will be present one day after exercising.
- Swelling in the back of the foot that may be present constantly but worsens through the day with activity.
- A pop sound at the back of the ankle can indicate a partial or complete rupture of the Achilles tendon.

Osteoarthritis

Arthritis of the Knee Joint

- Joint pain and stiffness may be present.
- Swelling of the affected joint may be present.
- Crepitations can be felt on the movement of the affected joint.
- There will be a loss of muscle strength.
- The range of movement will be reduced in the joint.
- Symptoms of joint pain are usually worse in the mornings.
- Redness and tenderness present in the affected joint.
- Patients can experience difficulty in walking and buckling of the affected knee joint.

Arthritis of the Hip Joint

- Pain, swelling, and tenderness may be present in the affected hip joint.
- Pain may be stabbing and sharp, or it may present with a dull ache.
- Joint stiffness is present when getting out of bed in the morning or after sitting for a prolonged time.
- Inability to bend down and perform routine activities.
- Pain in the thigh or the buttock on the affected side.
- Patients may experience difficulty in walking.
- Stiffening of the hip joint is present.

Chronic Pain Conditions

Fibromyalgia

- Widespread pain that is described as a constant dull ache lasting for more than three months.
- The pain will be present on both sides of the body, below and above the waist.
- Chronic feeling of tiredness despite sleeping for long hours.
- Associated sleep disorders such as sleep apnea and restless leg syndrome may be present.
- Patient has poor ability to focus or concentrate, a condition referred to as 'fibro fog.'
- Tenderness on palpation of at least 11 of the 18 recognized tender points.
- Patients can have associated chronic fatigue syndrome, anxiety, or depression.

Trigger Points (Myofascial Pain Syndrome)

- Deep aching muscle pain will be present.
- The pain will be persistent and can worsen with time.
- Muscle knot that is painful to touch will be present.

- The pain can worsen when the affected muscle is stretched or strained.
- Sleep difficulties due to the constant pain.
- Referred pain can also occur where pressure on a sensitive point can cause pain in an unrelated part of the body.
- Numbness and weakness of muscles can be present.
- Movement can be restricted or limited in the adjoining joints.

Chronic Headaches

Trigeminal Neuralgia
- Numbness or a tingling sensation in the cheek and jaw area.
- There can be short-lived bursts of severe pain.
- Pain may also present as jolts of stabbing or electrical type pain.
- Episodes of pain may be triggered by activities such as chewing or talking.
- Burning sensation present all over the face.
- Symptoms may be set off by touching the face for reasons such as shaving, washing, and putting on make-up.
- A strong wind blowing on the face can also trigger pain at times.
- Patients can experience a refractory period after one paroxysmal attack of pain where a new attack cannot be initiated.
- The pain is seen to worsen over time in some people.
- Sometimes patients experience long periods of remission.

Migraine
- Intense pain in the head.
- Throbbing or pulsing sensation in one or multiple sides of the head.

- Nausea and vomiting.
- Sensitivity to light and sound.
- Symptom progression usually follows the pattern of prodrome, aura, attack, and post-drome.
- Prodrome: Sensitivity to light, sound or smell, fatigue, food cravings, mood changes, severe thirst, etc.
- Aura: Black dots, wavy lines, tunnel vision, heavy feeling in arms and legs, ringing in the ears, tingling and numbness on one side of the body, and changes in smell, taste, or touch.
- Attack: Dull ache grows into throbbing pain. Pain worsens with physical activity. Pain can move from one side of the head to the other. Associated nausea and vomiting may be present.
- Post-drome: Patients either feel tired, wiped out, and cranky or unusually refreshed and happy. Muscle pain and weakness may be present.

I believe that this symptom guide can help you easily identify the possible conditions that you or one of your loved ones might be suffering from. Your healthcare provider or orthopedician can then perform the necessary clinical examinations, clinical tests, and investigations to narrow down the exact diagnosis.

Accurate treatment provided at the right time can help relieve pain and restore function to a great extent. We have seen in the preceding chapters that chronic pain can be avoided in most disease conditions if the correct treatment measures are instituted early in a proper manner.

The doctor has to diagnose accurately and the patient has to be willing to follow the doctor's advice completely for getting the maximum benefits of any therapy. However, prevention is the best medicine. Following a healthy lifestyle can ensure that you do not develop any of these diseases in the first place.

CONCLUSION

Pain always has a story. Whether it is physical or mental pain, there is always a cause, and the trick is to find it or recognize it. That is the route to lasting healing. As you read through the different chapters of this book, this concept would have been clear to you. However, let me explain with an example.

Mahesh was brought up entirely by his hard-working mother. His father had abandoned the family when he was just a little boy, and his mother eked out a living as a daily wage earner. Owing to the innumerable hardships he suffered, Mahesh was always a quiet, morose boy. Eventually, when he started working in a private company, he was unable to relate to his co-workers or make any meaningful friendships. He realized that he was harboring a lot of bitterness inside him. He finally sought professional help at the age of 35, and this helped him realize the chronic pain of abandonment that he had been carrying inside for all these years. He understood that this chronic pain in his mind had made him bitter and kept him from living life to the fullest.

This holds true for all of us—there is always a root cause for pain of any kind. This is the message that I seek to convey to my readers. It is important to understand and identify the root cause of the pain before the condition can be managed with correct diagnosis and a multidisciplinary approach.Our journey at Alleviate is all about generating a behavioral change in people toward chronic pain. This would include the patients receiving care as well as the healthcare providers. Pain management per se is a beautiful specialty and deserves more awareness among the people. There can be nothing more rewarding for a healthcare provider than to relieve a sufferer's pain, and for a patient with chronic pain, to finally become pain-free. Increased awareness can indeed create this behavioral change whereby people with chronic pain would choose to go to a pain clinic rather than to big hospitals where they were likely to run up huge hospital bills for admission and treatment.

My hope is that this book will convey the deep-seated role of interventional pain management and regenerative therapy in society. This has already been understood by the people in Western countries, where these therapies have been helping patients overcome pain for the last three to four decades. It is about time that this specialty and these therapies get their recognition in our country as well, and people see their positive impact on the quality of life.

The secret to managing chronic pain lies in taking one small step at a time but being consistent about it. The aim could be to decrease pain, reduce body weight, increase muscle strength, or overall rehabilitation. People need to understand that anything that has been wrong for a long period cannot get better all of a sudden. It takes a step-by-step, day-by-day approach. And this approach increases the chance of success phenomenally. If this book helped you or your loved ones live a pain-free life, then I would say my efforts have borne fruit.

ABOUT THE AUTHOR

Dr. Swagatesh Bastia [MBBS, MS (Ortho), Fellow in Trauma and Orthopaedics, UK] is the co-founder of Alleviate Pain Management Clinic, a chain of pain clinics in Bangalore specializing in treating chronic pain conditions.

Dr. Bastia is a qualified Orthopedic Surgeon. After completing his Master's in Orthopedics from Chennai, he underwent training in Endospine Surgery under Dr. PC Dey at the AMRI Hospital, Bhubaneshwar. Dr. Bastia also has completed Fellowship in Trauma and Orthopaedics at King's College Hospital, London. Dr. Bastia has spent two years of his life traveling across Europe and America and has a deep understanding of how Interventional Pain Management and Regenerative Medicine are bringing about a positive difference in innumerable people's lives. He has applied the same principles and standards at Alleviate.

Dr. Bastia believes that no one should live in pain, and it is his aim to make people aware of how they can lead a better and pain-free life.